GODS, HEROES AND GROUPS

GODS, HEROES AND GROUPS
Relational Dynamics through Mythic Archetypes

Brant Elwood & Aodhán Moran

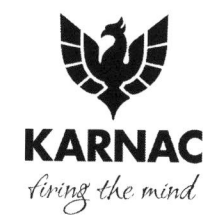

KARNAC
firing the mind

First published in 2025 by
Karnac Books Limited
62 Bucknell Road
Bicester
Oxfordshire OX26 2DS

British Library Cataloguing in Publication Data

A C.I.P. for this book is available from the British Library

ISBN: 978-1-80013-287-0 (paperback)
ISBN: 978-1-80013-288-7 (e-book)
ISBN: 978-1-80013-289-4 (PDF)

Typeset by Medlar Publishing Solutions Pvt Ltd, India

www.firingthemind.com

Contents

About the authors

Brant Elwood has an MA in Social-Organisational Psychology from Columbia University and is a therapeutic consultant. He has held leadership positions within several therapeutic treatment organisations. During the pandemic, he directed a non-profit that utilised myth and archetypal theory to conduct rites of passage work with young men in the southeast US.

Brant draws from the mythopoetic lineage of Robert Bly, Robert Johnson, and others in an attempt to establish a novel style of thinking about groups in communities and organisations. He first attended a Tavistock-style group relations conference in 2015.

Aodhán Moran has one foot in psychology and the other in technology. Starting his career in tech and e-commerce, Aodhán worked various roles in start-ups and scale-ups across Galway, San Francisco, and Toronto before pursuing a career in clinical psychology.

Aodhán is a certified executive coach through Dr Simon Western's Eco-Leadership Institute. His practice is grounded in the analytic-network systems psychodynamic lens, which he uses to coach young entrepreneurs toward self-awareness in their work.

As a student of group relations since 2019, Aodhán has attended multiple group relations-style conferences in member, trainee consultant, and staff roles, including The Tavistock Institute of Human Relations' Leicester Conference. Aodhán draws on Carl Jung, Joseph Campbell, Jonathan Pageau, René Girard, Simon Western, and others in his explorations of individual and group dynamics.

Aodhán is particularly interested in the intersection of psychology, mythology, and religion, and how these areas can inform our understanding of individual and group behaviour.

Foreword

Dear reader,

You are about to embark on a journey that I hope is the first in a series. This text by Brant and Aodhán is the material of our time and it is my wish that this will lead on to further, deeper exchanges.

It is now 2024 and we are facing war on every continent, brutality, greed, and corruption at every level of social, political, cultural, and spiritual systems. We need a new set of narratives and ways into understanding what has brought us here, and what may help us make a new road.

Through the lens of mythos, Brant and Aodhán have opened a vista for new sight and a capacity for new thought about our social ills and compulsions. This book looks at myths across cultures and historical periods and enters a realm of imaginal narrative in which the contents of the collective unconscious can be seen and connected to the reader, wherever they are in space and time.

In order to engage in a balanced, harmonious future, we need people and systems to be able to hold the complexity of our social field and revisit our mythical matrix—moving beyond the binary and reconciling ourselves as integrated Mythic-Beings.

It is a long Hero's Journey for all of us, and this text is a vital map on our way. This book is a welcome text to help us put ourselves back together.

Dr Leslie Brissett
Group Relations Programme Director at the Tavistock Institute of
Human Relations, 2017–2023

Introduction

How does a Norse creation myth warn us about obstacles that groups face during their forming phase?

How can Odysseus' escape from the Cyclops inform modern leaders about navigating the mob mentality within a group?

We wrote this book because we wanted to read it, and it did not exist. Advice about group dynamics and leadership is plentiful, as is the application of mythology to personal psychology. Yet the application of mythology to modern group psychology seems to be largely unexplored territory. Both authors contributed to every chapter in this text, but some of the experiences in organisations belong to one or the other. When not specifically noted, the use of 'I' refers to Brant's first-person perspective.

We hope to introduce a different approach to conceptualising groups; an approach that investigates group psychology through the lens of mythology. We wrote it for anyone interested in building a better understanding of group processes—leaders, therapists, and group facilitators may find it especially applicable.

Interpretive work of any kind is more of an art than a science, and this may be especially true when we focus on groups instead of individuals.

As a result, there is a level of open-mindedness and tolerance to mystery required from you, the reader.

This type of work asks us to indulge in the dramatic, since the mythic storytelling elements possess a certain grandeur. Marion Woodman (1998) speaks to the function and necessity of grand metaphor in *Sitting by the Well*. In short, metaphorical connections amplify the meaning we imbue into our experiences.

Myths seem to capture patterns of the universal human experience, and this is because they deal with archetypes. Popularised by Jung, archetypes are inherited psychobiological structures common to all of humanity. Joseph Campbell (1949) wrote his mega-hit, *The Hero with a Thousand Faces*, because he perceived the same Hero archetype across different historical periods. Campbell observes its manifestation in ancient epics, folklore, and the lives of great religious heroes like Gautama Śakyamūni and Christ, as well as within case notes of modern psychiatric patients. These archetypal patterns are brought to life as gods, demigods, heroes, and Titans in our favourite mythological stories.

I (Brant) have always been impressed with certain colleagues' ability to connect the seemingly mundane to the mythical. A skilled therapist might say of a client: 'His story is the Icarus myth. His parents haven't held boundaries, he parties until 3 am, and he's ended up in the hospital twice from overdose. He flies too close to the sun, and our work here is to ground him in an identity that allows him to keep his feet on the earth and get a sense for limits'.

As Woodman (1998) states, the application of mythic metaphor takes things to a deeper, more meaningful level, into the realm of the psychological archetype. A curtain is pulled away, and the possibility of deeper self-knowledge and richer associations becomes apparent. We touch something ancient and primal when mythology is brought into the mundane.

Another distinct skill that I admire in colleagues is the ability to manage complex group dynamics and steer groups towards productive ends. In wilderness therapy, where I began my career, most clients attend involuntarily and carry anger and resentment as a result. Many bring a history of intense maladaptive behaviour, and all of them have extensive defence mechanisms in place. Yet somehow, the best therapists and field instructors consistently get extraordinary outcomes. Skilful facilitation enables these groups to hold emotionally safe environments that allow connection and sharing at a deep level. With the right guidance, the group becomes greater than the sum of its parts.

During graduate school, I was introduced to the group relations work of the Tavistock tradition. Group relations conferences usually last three to five days, and instead of lecture formats, they involve visceral interrelational experiences. Most of the time spent at a conference centres around the task of assessing the group dynamics as they arise. It is difficult to explain such an experiential process in words, but there are two defining characteristics of group relations work that changed my perspective on understanding groups.

The orientation of the work assumes a group-as-a-whole lens. This means that we accept that the group has a mind of its own, and that understanding the group psyche (especially the unconscious) is the goal. Further, this means that individuals' actions are assumed to mean something about the group, first and foremost. We avoid indulging in explanations for behaviour that focus on an individual's motivations. If a member leaves to go to the bathroom during a session, for example, the assumption is that this means something about the group-as-a-whole. Some part of the group wanted to flee the room, perhaps. We can be agnostic to this concept and still benefit from the process. The idea is to suspend disbelief and ask, 'What if the group has a mind of its own that is pulling the strings? How does this individual's action serve the group-as-a-whole?' The value of this becomes clearer with practice.

The work is done in the here-and-now. The task is to analyse the group dynamics 'in the room' as they are happening. This means that politics, childhood struggles, or outside persons are only relevant as they relate to a dynamic currently in the room. This practice leaves most participants feeling naked, in a sense. Group members cannot hide as easily behind past stories of themselves, or the distractions of broader society. In group relations work, the facilitators (consultants) confront the group when the group moves to topics that are not 'in the room'. For example, in groups that find themselves constantly bringing up politics from the outside, a consultant might remark to the group, 'This group seems to enjoy the fantasy that they can run away from difficulties in the room by uniting around a dislike of Donald Trump. I wonder what it is that is hard to look at in this group right now'. The group has the choice to take this comment up for discussion or not, of course, and each option says something about the inner workings of the group-as-a-whole.

I left my first conference feeling angry and indignant, but I realised that anything that could offend me could also teach me, and I attended my second conference one year later. This work spurred an 'Aha!' moment for me, as I began to look at groups in a different light and started asking different questions. I started to observe the subtle ways that groups use individuals, and the unwritten contracts to which individuals adhere when they join groups. Nuanced roles develop, and behaviour changes drastically for individuals as they step into these roles. A heightened sense of these underlying forces is a kind of superpower for any group member, especially for someone in a leadership role.

Both mythic interpretation and group relations work serve to expand our understanding of the psyche. What happens when we examine group dynamics through a mythological lens?

CHAPTER 1

The group effect

In the wilderness of the Appalachian Mountains, a group of adolescent boys breaks down camp and prepares to hike. This is a wilderness therapy programme, and none of the boys have elected to be here. Yet, overall, the camaraderie is strong between the eight young men and their four field instructors. They have everything they need on their backs, and the quality of their day will depend on the effort they put in.

The group starts the day off strong—all except for Sam. For the fourth day in a row, Sam shuts down and refuses to do chores, eat, or drink. Group members begin to grumble among themselves, 'Here we go again'.

Sam's refusal will impact the group. If he does not hike, they will have to set camp back up and stay at the same site, where they have been stuck for the past four days, which none of them want. The instructors try to contain the discontent of the group members as they glare in Sam's direction. It seems that everyone agrees that Sam is the problem in the group, and that if he were gone, the group would function at a higher level.

After two more days of this—and heightening tension between the group and Sam—he ends up leaving the programme for medical reasons. The group is ecstatic. The boys play games, joke around, and prepare to hike out of camp. Everyone has the impression that the group is on the verge of building a strong culture and becoming a real team.

This feeling lasts about two hours.

As the students approach the new campsite, Jesse—a student who had been respectful, cooperative, and relatively dependable up to that point—begins to emotionally escalate. There is no obvious trigger; the group had done a hike of medium difficulty in the heat, and it is reasonable for any of the guys to feel homesick, but the timing is certainly strange. He throws a tantrum and begins making threats about walking off into the woods, and two staff are pulled over to sit with him.

In the blink of an eye, the group has a new Sam, and the members resume their grumbling and blaming. Jesse, who had been fairly reasonable previously, remains uncharacteristically belligerent, and this becomes the new normal over the next days.

An instructor mutters, 'This group is haunted'.

Leaders and experienced professionals who work with teams may relate to this scenario. What happened here? From the field instructor perspective, is it a matter of identifying and correcting the individual problems of Sam and Jesse, or might there be a deeper way of interpreting the situation?

Groups are complicated, and there is likely not a single simple answer that we can ever arrive at with full confidence. We could attempt to explain Sam and Jesse's behaviour separately from the group context, but we might also consider what effect the group itself had.

The word *group* is not sexy, but perhaps it should be. Groups exert a powerful effect on individual behaviour, an effect that is typically underappreciated and misunderstood. The phrase 'a group of humans' has much deeper implications than 'a group of buildings'.

Within this book, we will define a group as more than two people who share a mutual and interdependent interest in at least one specific goal. This includes organisations, teams, businesses, and even society. This also includes a group of people riding a bus. It may not feel like a coherent group, but there are some common goals for passengers; namely, arriving at the destination safely.

Groups exist like Russian dolls, nested within each other. The specific group we identify with at any given moment depends on the circumstances. As I write, I am conscious of being an American, a man, a director for a men's recovery programme, and a resident of Asheville. However, if circumstances highlighted other parts of my identity, my mind would switch gears accordingly. For example, when I hear spoken Mandarin, I recall my days as an expatriate in Chengdu and the student group to which I belonged at the time. The groups with which we most clearly identify during a given moment are dictated by the confluence of our total self-narrative and the context. We all contain within ourselves many stories of identity. The situation determines which of our stories come into play.

On a larger scale, and similarly, societies have stories about themselves and the world as well. Although many new stories are written and adopted, there is something powerful and profound about the old stories that have shaped so much of culture and stayed with us through the ages—the myths. We can hypothesise that they communicate something important about the shared human experience. The application to the individual psyche has been explored by thinkers such as Freud, Jung, Marie-Louise von Franz, Robert Bly, Robert Johnson, Joseph Campbell, Marion Woodman, and others. Yet we see a dearth of mythic interpretation at a group dynamics level at a time when such insight could provide much value.

We do not mean to suggest that ancient myths were consciously intended to speak about human group dynamics, *per se*. Yet the human unconscious expresses deeper archetypal truths through our stories, and these can be applied to illuminate both the individual and the group psyche. Simply put, these stories are treated as a gateway to the unconscious. The result is that we can draw thought-provoking parallels between themes in mythology and our modern study of groups.

One style of interpreting myth holds that each character in a story represents a piece of the self, and thus any myth is contained within the psyche (or group psyche, in this case). Following this line of thought, myths are not accounts of the past, but accounts of within. Therefore, when myths are narrated here, we use the present tense. The Villain, the Hero, the Mentor, and the Victim all reside inside our 'interior kingdom' in the now. With the group dynamics lens in place, this means that all elements or characters within a myth represent elements of the group psyche.

This work is exploratory and interpretive in nature, and not an exhaustive investigation by any means. Astute readers will notice that the themes we have picked out are not distinct, as there is significant overlap between concepts. The frameworks and myths drawn from here are somewhat cherry-picked based on limitations of our own intellect, cultural biases, and current understanding of groups. We view this as a starting point, and hopefully a fruitful introduction for readers to synthesise myth and the study of groups.

We invite you to join us in suspending disbelief and adopting two assumptions that will aid the creative process. The first is that there are no coincidences in myth. Every character and detail has relevant meaning. Every action implies something deeper and greater than what may appear on the surface.

The second assumption is that there are no coincidences in group behaviour.

CHAPTER 2

A little bit of theory: Projection and projective identification

Before going further, there is a pair of helpful concepts we can pull from psychology literature: projection and projective identification.

As humans, it is natural that we feel more comfortable with some parts of ourselves than others. We may enjoy our sense of humour or dislike our quick temper. We are conditioned by those around us at an early age to accentuate some parts of our personality, and repress or tightly control the rest. To be human is to endure this process, since the approval of our caretakers and peers determines survival when we are infants. It is not a process anyone skips; although the style and efficacy of our caregivers matter. Nor do such pressures cease when we reach adulthood, although our mature awareness and relative independence may act as mitigating factors.

As a result of this process, we come to consider some parts of ourselves as unacceptable, and may be unwilling to even acknowledge them. The Jungians call this disowned psychic material 'shadow', and Robert Bly (1986) gives us a metaphor of a bag that we carry behind us, filled with the pieces of ourselves we have learned to stow away. We can pack them away, so to speak, but this psychic material never ends up going far. Repressed energies still want to find a way to be expressed, because they are a part of our humanness. As a result, a process called projection can occur.

Projection was discussed by Freud, and then Jung, von Franz, and others. It is the process of disowning a part of our psyche and displacing it onto another. In essence, we 'send out' a part of ourselves that is not integrated into our idea of who we are. We hand these qualities to another, imagining them to exist strongly and exclusively in this other person. The other is made to hold our baggage. It is a splitting of the psyche on a subconscious level.

When that projection is accepted by the other, or 'taken in', *projective identification* has occurred (Klein, 1946). If you remind one of your subordinates of their father, and they have not integrated that paternal energy, they begin to think of you as owning those qualities. They may feel resentful, or intimidated, or perhaps more relaxed, depending on their relationships early on in life. There is an unconscious invitation for you to then start acting in a more and more paternal manner. You both enter into an enmeshed relational dance if you 'accept' the invitation. These concepts are related to the ideas of transference and countertransference used in therapeutic literature (Stokoe, 2021).

These are not phenomena relegated to those with mental illness; it is something we all do every day, in subtle and not-so-subtle ways. Projections reveal themselves when the light shines just right; for example, when we call our boss 'dad' or 'mum' by mistake right before a big meeting, implying that our own paternal or maternal qualities are being *outsourced*. Slips of the tongue reveal much of our inner psychic architecture.

We project for reasons of unconscious self-protection. The inner racist, the inner bully, perhaps the inner weakling; it feels threatening to acknowledge these parts of ourselves, and so we project them outward for someone else to possess on our behalf. For the admirable qualities we refuse to own, we may feel unprepared to shoulder the responsibility that these qualities would demand of us. If I put my 'brilliance' in a teammate at work, I am off the hook for coming up with innovative ideas. Nathaniel Branden discusses this phenomenon in his *Six Pillars of Self-Esteem* (1995). Of course, this does not mean that others never possess such qualities, or that the claim here is that all perception is simply projection. There is room between our ears for both accurate assessment of others and projection. Yet it can be nearly impossible to differentiate between the two with confidence, and in this work, we err on the side of assuming projection to be at play in most cases.

Since the 'holders' of our projections are doing something important for us on a psychic level, we tend to be fiercely defensive of our projections. We will set up the holder of our psychic material to validate our expectations, and we may ignore information that contradicts them. We become attached to seeing them a certain way.

When strong emotion comes up, oftentimes it is a clue about our projections, if we know how to look. We should be especially suspicious of the situations that bring up anger in us; anger is a common way that we dim the light of awareness and keep our projections in place. Likewise, that which is considered taboo in groups is typically a rich place to focus exploration, with the understanding that we are treading on dangerous ground. That which offends us reveals us. One definition for revelation is 'the act of revealing', and proper personal work or group dynamics work should always have this quality. We should be celebrating the offensive quality of the work around projections. Psychic maturity involves reintegrating the shadowy parts of ourselves and our groups and processing the shame around each piece we have given away. It is not a fast process, and it is certainly painful at times.

CHAPTER 3

Creation myths and early group stages

In the mid-1960s, Bruce Tuckman (1965) contributed a model of group stages that is still widely cited today. It is a simple model that is easy to apply, and as a starting point it can help shed some light on how groups work. He contended that all groups progress through certain developmental stages: forming, storming, norming, performing, and adjourning (this last was a later addition). Any team goes through a similar trajectory, be it corporate executives or a Viking longboat crew. We might consider it an abbreviated 'Hero's Journey' for groups, for those familiar with Joseph Campbell's work.

Within Tuckman's model, we can expect that all groups need time for member relationships to develop (forming), differences to be explored and navigated (storming), and baseline etiquette to be embraced (norming), before we can expect a team to produce great work (performing). This is a simple application, but already we can draw the conclusion that a good leader needs to act in ways that facilitate the progression through these stages. A savvy leader sets appropriate expectations and tasks for the group based on where the group sits on the model at any given moment.

Of course, a model like this is merely the tip of the iceberg. Models give us a template for simplifying and understanding a complex world.

Identifying that a group is in the 'forming stage' conveys certain information, yet even the forming process itself is complex, and the mere recognition of a group stage may not give us enough actionable insight. But it is a way we can chunk down the world and start to prioritise which pieces of information we grace with our attention, and it is a good place to start to apply our mythic lens.

Like our psychology models, mythology also gives us templates for making meaning in a complex world. As we will see, we can find interesting points of confluence between ancient myth and modern group models. If Tuckman's model offers a simple starting point for learning about organisational psychology, creation myths offer an intuitive starting point from the mythic side. If myths are a map of the soul, then it stands to reason that creation myths say something about how we as humans form groups. After all, what are creation myths if not a *forming* of sorts?

Again, myths are grandiose, and their comparison to group processes may feel overdramatic at times. The dramatic element is helpful. It connects us to meaningful archetypes that we can use as metaphors in our more mundane group experiences of everyday life and work.

Let's start with the Norse creation myth:

> Creation begins with a void that sits between two extremes. To the north, there is a land of ice called Niflheim. In the south, there is a land of fire called Muspelheim. Eventually, the heat from the south melts some ice in the north. The melted ice from Niflheim forms the frost giant Ymir, the first being. As the flames warm the glaciers, Ymir's sweat spawns the race of giants, and a giant cow is created to feed the giants. The cow feeds on salt contained in the melting ice.

We are painted a picture of opposing polarities that are each inhospitable in different ways. This is a nice representation of the dilemma presented to individuals during the forming stage of a new group. Joining any new group starts with a double-bind for the individual, meaning that any choice presents significant drawbacks. Expanding on Klein's theories, Wilfred Bion (1959) claimed that individuals who are joining a group have to balance a fear of being consumed by the group, on one hand, with a fear of being rejected by the group, on the other (p. 91).

To lean into the group too fully is to be consumed by the southern flames of Muspelheim. We can associate the flames with passion, intimacy, and connection: experiences that bring joy when in balance, yet can incur a terrible price if unchecked. To be 'burned by the fire' is to lose one's sense of individual identity, to be merged fully with the group, as Wilfred Bion warns. Individuality is at risk of being consumed by the powerful group mind.

The opposite but equal threat is the northern ice. To be left out in the cold is a death sentence, written in our genetic code by ancestors who depended on the shared campfire for connection, warmth, and protection. The individual who remains 'only an individual' when the group forms is apt to be left out in the cold. In Mesopotamian lore, the Wild Man Enkidu says to Gilgamesh, 'Two people, companions, they can prevail together against the terror', as they fight with the demon Humbaba (Ferry, 1993). The world contains dangers, and the group provides protection. And yet, physical safety is not the full story. Wilfred Bion (1959) discussed what he believed is a distinct human need for grouping: 'I consider that group mental life is essential to the full life of the individual, quite apart from any temporary or specific need, and that satisfaction of this need has to be sought through membership of a group' (p. 56).

On the other hand, we can associate the ice with solitude, contemplation, and preservation. Again, there is importance in these experiences in the proper context (such as setting boundaries), and also there are deadly consequences when they are out of balance. Solitude, contemplation, and preservation may ferment into loneliness, rumination, and stagnation. Rejection from the group is as damaging as losing oneself to the group, and all individuals stepping into a new group membership must navigate these two threats.

In the *Odyssey*, Odysseus and his men have to pass through a treacherous strait that contains two monsters, Scylla and Charybdis. If the ship veers too close to the cliffs, Scylla plucks and kills individual men from the group. On the other hand, if they steer too far from the cliffs into the open water, the whole ship is pulled into a deadly whirlpool created by Charybdis.

Marion McCollum Hampton writes:

> Essentially, a large part of group dynamics literature proposes
> that group membership evoked the strong, contradictory wishes

that individual members have had in response to their mothers: on the one hand, to be fused with and indistinguishable from her; on the other, to be distinct and differentiated from her ... Individuals fear being swallowed up and lost in that undifferentiated mass; on the other hand, they fear the isolation and abandonment of being left out or rejected. (Gabriel & Hampton, 1999)

We can say that the formation of groups involves navigating questions around identity, among other things. How can an individual hold both their own identity and that of the group simultaneously? What happens when the identities of the self and that of the group member demand conflicting actions of the individual?

We can conclude that a healthy individual approaches a group with an engaged scepticism. We might also say that a healthy group allows for and encourages members to find a balance that preserves both the group and the individual. The temperature, so to speak, should not be too hot or too cold. In *Group Psychology and the Analysis of the Ego*, Freud (1921b) introduces us to Schopenhauer's porcupine metaphor: In the snow, a group of porcupines crowds together to keep warm, yet when they get too close, they accidentally stick each other, which causes them to jump back apart, until they become cold again, and so on. Some intimacy is life-giving, yet enmeshment causes injury. Too much fire or ice causes catastrophe.

Many of the more disastrous episodes in recent history have been well documented and illustrate the pitfalls. The Salem witch hunters, consumed by the southern flames, murdered their own community members. The Russian military police and citizens that allowed the Gulag to exist were seduced by the group identity as well. The faux prison guards of the Stanford Prison Experiment and the bankers who followed a system into economic ruin in 2008 share this in common. Yet, it is not just in the extreme periphery that we find this phenomenon. The seduction to lose oneself to a group identity exerts a force on all of us on a daily basis, in the form of self-censorship and pleaser patterns. We make small deals often that sacrifice individual expression for group harmony.

On the other end, the typical school shooter has been left to the northern ice. If accounts are to be believed, aloneness and alienation are strongly experienced by many of these individuals. Overexposure to the northern ice is also a contributing factor for those who 'act in', taking their own lives or performing acts of self-harm. More warmth and connection is needed.

Interestingly, the general public expresses a similar sentiment towards both the outcast and the totally enmeshed member of a toxic group. That is, the common response is harsh judgement. No one likes to consider that they might have indeed cooperated with the Nazi party's decrees under the right conditions, or that they might be capable of violence as a result of group rejection. Perhaps the poles of the continuum are less far apart than they first appear. Or perhaps, when the illusion is fully in place that only *those people over there* are the problem, some part of us believes we can attach a generic judgement to such unfortunate cases and be done with it. This is projection in action.

Despite our attempts to disown our susceptibility to group forces, the 'fire and ice' exert gravity upon us in every social situation. It is not something *out there*, it is something *in here*. It is not a matter of 'if', it is a matter of how aware we are of the effects. The Stanford Prison Experiment example is enjoyable precisely because it demonstrates the susceptibility to these forces of some of our most intelligent members of society. Every time we join a new work team, these forces are navigated, usually unconsciously. And often poorly.

Returning to the myth, we see that sustenance becomes available when the southern flames contact the northern ice. The giants only come to life when the frost giant Ymir experiences the heat. There is sweat, so we conclude that there is discomfort involved in the encounter. Indeed, preserving one's identity while navigating the forming stage of a group is hard work.

At the onset, the Norse people personify the icy end of the spectrum. The icy cold may be barbaric and treacherous in its own way, but it is the first to merit a name and hold human form. The group-as-a-whole, on the other hand, may be felt as the immolator of identity in the initial stages. We can visualise a burning pit that will singe our eyebrows off should we take a peek into its depths. Yet in the myth, contact with the warmth is required for life to populate the void. Likewise, we as individuals cannot remain fully independent of group forces and experience our full humanity.

We return to our myth:

> The gods are then born from the giants—Odin, Vili, and Ve—who rise up to murder Ymir, the original frost giant. Most of the other giants drown in Ymir's blood as it falls. Ymir's body is used to create the Earth and Heavens.

The Norse had a penchant for the graphic. Not only did Ymir die, but most of the other giants drowned in his blood. Referencing Tuckman's model, we can imagine that this imagery corresponds to the storming phase. Storming involves a renegotiation of roles, group norms, and the power structure. When new groups form, it is quite common that the first person to assume leadership is scapegoated or 'killed off' in some fashion. We discuss this in further detail in the next chapters—but it is worth touching on briefly now.

This death often manifests as tacit disempowerment handed down by the group-as-a-whole, but could also mean a member leaving the system, or even literal assassination. For this reason, seasoned leaders or coaches of groups often refrain from taking a central leadership role as a new group forms. Although stepping into immediate leadership may be seductive, it is generally not the skilled approach in groups without explicit hierarchies. The Ymirs are typically deposed. The second wave of leaders to rise up often has more staying power. In these mythic frameworks—and in my experiences with group relations work—the first mouse triggers the mousetrap, the second mouse gets the cheese. There is more information available about emergent group values and norms at this point. 'Patience is a virtue' becomes actionable advice.

A group is motivated by certain unconscious drives in its initial forming phase, and these priorities shift as the initial forming is accomplished. Leaders who serve the group well with forming tasks may not provide for the group's desires as they move into a new stage. Perhaps the personalities that ease the anxiety in the beginning and allow bonding cannot serve the group with more complex tasks.

We conclude our myth with the introduction of humans:

> As Ymir decomposed, the dwarves were made from the maggots consuming Ymir's body. Other gods arose to join the original three,

and Asgard was established as their home. Only then were humans created.

The Norse tell us that dwarves precede humans. We might associate dwarves with toughness, building, and boundaries. They are foundational. In a practical sense, this means that there is work to be done 'before the humans arrive'. Humanness is sometimes equated with vulnerability, emotionality, and imperfection. When a top athlete is humbled in competition, announcers say that s/he 'looks human'. Exposing too much of the 'humanness' in the early stages of group formation amounts to humans intruding on the dwarves' time.

We may encounter an overly expressive person at a party who shares about their relationship with their mother before proper introductions and small talk have happened. It feels premature when someone spills their soul into the room so early. Boundaries have not been navigated yet, nor group norms established, and these steps should not be skipped—that is 'dwarf work'. True human vulnerability is a rare feat for groups to achieve, and there is groundwork required beforehand. Most groups never arrive there, and most group tasks do not demand it.

The group usually has mechanisms in place to extinguish or transmute oversharing behaviour in nascent stages. This person may be an early candidate for a group scapegoat, for example. They may serve the group by 'being the awkward one', and allowing others to relax, knowing that they themselves will not be asked to hold the awkwardness for the group.

An overarching theme here is that both group stages and creation myths offer a somewhat linear storyline. The rules may not be entirely fixed and sequential, but there is a sense of order to the events. Leaders and group members often intuitively feel this, and it is wise to consider this in our dealings with groups.

CHAPTER 4

Hierarchies and power in groups

Tuckman's stages are not controversial, *per se*, but other concepts discussed in this work are. The concept of hierarchy, for example, has taken on a strong emotional charge in our current cultural context. It is often said that Millennials and Gen Z tend to be averse to crystallised hierarchy in the workplace. In a leadership role I took with a therapeutic centre, I was handed an organisational chart that only included names and departments, without indicating any sense of power differentiation. Robert Bly warns us of this developing cultural orientation in his book *The Sibling Society* (Bly, 1997).

Yet in mythology, hierarchies are widespread in stories across different cultures. We see gods presiding over humans, and even among the gods there is typically a pecking order. Regardless of our comfort level with the topic, power dynamics are woven into the fabric of our human stories. We can apply the logic Joseph Campbell used when drafting the Hero's Journey: If commonalities show up across cultures the world over, through different historical time periods, then they reflect something deep and archetypal within our shared psyche. Hierarchy and power differences were not invented by modern man. In this work, our goal is to acknowledge that force within groups and become curious about it. As a general rule, aversion to an archetypal force such as hierarchy leads to unhealthy repression; that is, a lack of integration.

Turning to mythology, we see a dynamic hierarchy established early on in the Greek pantheon.

> Uranus is born of Gaia, and then becomes her mate and equal. They give birth to the Titans, as well as three Cyclops and the fifty-headed beasts known as the Hecatoncheires. Uranus proves to be a harsh father, and his offspring come to hate and fear him. Cronus, the last-born, is the only Titan brave enough to attempt an overthrow, and when Uranus comes to lie with Gaia, Cronus ambushes him with a sickle, severing his genitals and casting them into the sea. Uranus either dies or is permanently exiled, but first he promises punishment for the Titans.
>
> Cronus marries his sister Rhea, and they give birth to the gods and goddesses. Since he fears being overthrown by his children, he swallows each of them upon birth, until a furious Rhea feeds him a stone instead of the sixth-born Zeus. Zeus grows up away from the Titans on Crete, and eventually returns to secretly feed a potion to Cronus, inducing him to vomit out the other gods, who are still alive. With their help, Zeus is able to conquer Cronus and send him into imprisonment in Tartarus, a vast realm of darkness under the Earth. After suppressing revolt attempts from the remaining Titans and other entities, Zeus reigns over creation, and holds the throne over the other gods and goddesses.

Zeus rules Olympus with his retinue of lower gods. Odin reigns in Norse mythology. Horus wins the throne from Set in Egypt. Anu is the head of the Babylonian gods. Huitzilopochtli holds prominence among Aztec deities. Though we can find examples of female deities holding hierarchical prominence, such as the Shinto sun goddess Amaterasu, we notice an over-representation of the masculine holding formal power among extant prominent myths. Feminine spirits are often given a care-taking role for the Earth: Pachamama of the Incas, Gaia of the Greeks, etc.

Setting aside politics and personal feelings, we might ask why so many cultures have manifested this. It seems that it has served the group-as-a-whole in some way to recruit the masculine energies for the ordered leadership role and the feminine energies for the nurtur-ing leadership role, with some exceptions. This does not imply men are better suited to lead than women, nor that men cannot be nurturing. It is evidence, however, that the collective psyche has a tendency to place masculine energies in positions of power, and there is always a 'why' for any group action such as this—often we see that these group tendencies are the manifestations of unconscious drives.

A group-as-a-whole explanation demands deeper insight than 'Men are power-hungry and disempower women', or 'Men are meant to be the leaders'. Both views are politically oriented and overly simplistic. They are also beside the point in the context of group dynamics study. Neither view applies a group-as-a-whole lens to help us gain a deeper understanding of the processes within the group psyche.

We have the evidence from the myths, and we assume the group psyche mobilises certain members to fill certain roles for a reason that serves the group. It would seem that members embodying the masculine archetypal energy often serve as more ready vessels for the group projections around leadership. The question is not 'Is mythol-ogy sexist?'; the question is 'What is it about our group-as-a-whole that tends to recruit masculine archetypes into leadership roles—or at least, the qualities that groups have historically associated with masculinity?'

It is a leader's responsibility to manoeuvre through this skilfully. Carl Jung believed that both men and women draw on masculine and feminine internal resources (Jung, 1969). Both men and women in leadership roles should be in touch with Zeus, Odin, or Horus, not because men are meant to rule, but because our groups are telling us about some of the qualities they need in leadership through the myths. Leaders can and sometimes should choose not to cooperate with group biases, but this choice is better made when tempered with an awareness of group unconscious patterns.

If hierarchies are inherent, then we must also acknowledge they are not static. The myths reveal a constantly shifting landscape of power differences, and we see the same in our own groups and organisations. It is hard to imagine a story at all without this dynamic quality. Themes of regicide and overthrow are commonplace in myth. Cronus castrates his father Uranus to take the throne, and Zeus rises up to take power from Cronus. Odin and the Norse gods are involved in many battles and misadventures with would-be revolutionary forces.

In the US, the anger towards the established power systems is palpable. There has been a recent political movement explicitly aimed at distributing power from the wealthiest 1 per cent (Bates et al., 2016). Most of our movies share the theme of the powerful villain who must be courageously overthrown by a heroic underdog. Through our modern stories, we reflect back animosity towards those in power, and a fascination with dethroning them. Regardless of the stated justifications for this, the group-as-a-whole lens tasks us to simply recognise that the group psyche manifests anger towards those in power, and perhaps even the idea of power. Again, we assume that this setup is serving an unconscious drive for the group on some level. There are internal revolutionary forces that have persisted across time and culture. We see signs of ambivalence—hierarchies are consistently manifested and consistently resented.

The resentment for those *above* seems to have a primordial rooting. In his book *The Science of Storytelling*, Will Storr (2019) asserts the archetypal nature of the narrative in which low-ranking characters conspire to topple the dominating powers above. Pulling from story theorist Christopher Booker, Storr argues that disorder at the top of a hierarchy is solved by regenerative activity at lower levels. The archetypal qualities typically associated with the feminine, then, become important pieces to integrate for any leader who wants to achieve longevity in their role. We see this theme repeated in chimpanzee alphas: their leadership is retained only by caring, protecting, and providing for those lower on the social ladder, keeping resentment at bay (De Waal, 2005). The unbalanced masculine is apt to manifest a beheading.

While it is certainly true that many hierarchies do not end up serving the people, one problem with outright dismantling the current system is that it betrays an arrogance about our understanding of groups and systems. Hierarchies are structures of power, so perhaps a structural metaphor will suffice: It is unwise to remove a load-bearing pillar from the living room—no matter how many times we have bumped our heads against it. We must understand something of the architecture of the house before we can act appropriately, lest we bring the whole thing down on ourselves. We need to be able to answer the questions, 'Why did the group create this for itself? What deeper drive exists?' Until we are confident in our ability to do so, it is often best to proceed with humble caution.

Is hierarchy inevitable?

Aodhán Moran

Lower Olympian gods and goddesses often transgress Zeus' authority, yet are still under his rule. Rebelling against authority suggests being 'ruled over', as it still occurs within the hierarchy, against a ruling force. As De Mello and Stroud (1990) noted, you are still tied with that which you renounce.

Although there are legitimate reasons to call for the dissolution of specific power structures, hierarchy is an inescapable component of group life. Humans are evolutionarily geared towards goal orientation, achievement of status, and competitive behaviours.

One style of thinking holds that functional hierarchy orients us in the world by defining us in relationship to the ideal on top. This ideal serves as a role model. In the domain we strive to achieve, we look upwards, and pattern our first attempts after the greats in the field. It is no mistake that the word *pattern* is rooted in the Latin *pater*, which means father.

Paul Moxnes (1999) echoes Jung and Freud in asserting that the archetypal structure of the organisation is the family. He postulates that seven archetypal roles strive to become real in culture, myth, groups, and organisations. He called these archetypes 'deep roles', going as far as to say that group life would degenerate into a collective psychosis without the ordering power of these archetypes (Figure 1). Primary deep roles stem from the basic traditional family unit, and include both positive and negative potentials:

- Father (Positive: King, Negative: Beast)
- Mother (Positive: Queen, Negative: Witch)
- Son (Positive: Prince, Negative: Black Sheep)
- Daughter (Positive: Princess, Negative: Whore)

Secondary deep roles include:

- Material Helper (Positive: Faithful Servant, Negative: Judas)
- Spiritual Helper (Positive: Wise Man, Negative: Pretender)
- Transformational Roles (Positive: Hero-Winner, Negative: Clown-Loser).

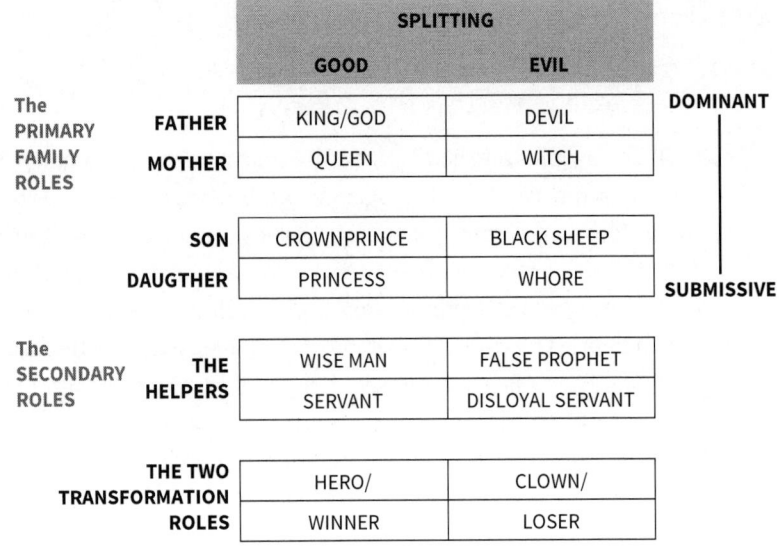

Figure 1. Deep role theory: a psychodynamic perspective on roles. (Based on Figure 2 in Moxnes, 1999. Reproduced with permission.)

Building on Jung, Moxnes (1999) claimed that deep roles are biologically mediated, yet socially constructed patterns of relating that strive to become real. Similar to the Muses in Ancient Greece, who possessed and did their work through the poets and playwrights, deep roles possess and do their work through group members. With a nod to Bion's basic assumptions of dependency, fight–flight, and pairing (Bion, 1959), we might say that the specific deep roles manifested by the group psyche speak to the current set of unmet psychological needs. The leadership qualities given most weight hint at what archetype is active in the group psyche.

If we imagine that a group is like an organism, then it follows that a hierarchy must promote psychic homeostasis—this is a core function of the structure of any group in a changing world.

Additionally, a general principle in depth psychology theory is that opposites call to each other to create balance. Carl Jung (1971) termed this phenomenon enantiodromia, which refers to the tendency of the unconscious opposite to emerge over time. This holds true in hierarchical systems. If a group repudiates authority, or if authority controls too tightly, an equally powerful counter-position builds up in the unconscious, and this energy will look for an opportunity for expression. Often, the psyche's efforts to restore equilibrium result in a violent swing towards the opposing disposition. Cronus ruled during a golden age without a need for law, yet he became oppressive towards his offspring until he was overthrown by Zeus. The hierarchy is not ever truly dismantled, it is simply transmuted, or inverted.

As referenced earlier, journalist Will Storr discusses the human tendency to root for the underdog and revolt against what is 'above'. And indeed, brain imaging studies show that brain regions associated with pleasure activate when watching high-status individuals fall from grace. A group's desire to protect the marginalised may be unconsciously driven by a desire to tear down those in authority, forming an inverted hierarchy—a 'hierarchy of the people'. This is possibly a more prominent feature of Western civilisation. We will discuss this a bit more in depth in the chapter on mythic murder.

CHAPTER 5

Leadership succession and worship

We conceptualise leadership as one's ability to influence a group towards a meaningful goal. Obholzer & Roberts (2019) would add that leadership implies followership from others. Leaders act as building blocks for the construction of hierarchy, and as such, the emergent qualities that are celebrated in leadership roles reveal much about the group-as-a-whole. Leadership is contextual and determined by the needs of the group. Through a group relations lens, we expect that leaders are pulled forward or summoned forth by the group psyche's rich cache of drives. This perspective runs counter to early Freudian thought about group dynamics, in which a leader was said to exercise strong willpower over an insipid crowd.

Taking a group lens means we need to pay special attention to the qualities summoned up into leadership roles by our groups of study. In some groups, we see a longing for an infallible saviour. The fantasy of an omnipotent, beneficent leader provides a sense of comfort—someone who has all the answers, and thus can unburden the group of the collective anxiety and responsibility of decision-making. In therapeutic groups, this role is often given to the therapist. In popular culture, we can see this manifested towards celebrities and political figures. Elon Musk is this for some, or Oprah, or Michelle Obama, or Trump. Wilfred Bion calls this unconscious drive *dependency*, and we could interpret this as a group fantasy to preserve infancy. In myth, we might see this phenomenon represented by the worship we see for certain deities. Which deity is worshipped, metaphorically, might give us clues as to what type of hierarchy might emerge.

Group-as-a-whole thinking also allows us to make some connections between leadership in myth and the stages of groups (forming, norming, etc.). We can ask the question: 'How does the group unconscious interact with the stages of groups to determine what type of leader will emerge?' It is possible, perhaps even implied, that the unconscious drives of the group shift as a group moves to a new stage of development. It also follows that a group would demand leadership qualities based on which unconscious drive is manifested in the current moment. This could explain why the Greek creation myth features a rapid succession from Uranus to Cronus, and then from Cronus to Zeus. The leader that served the group during its forming phase may not be deemed acceptable by the group as it transitions to the storming phase, and the group psyche will manifest a *coup d'état* when necessary to remedy this.

We see this enacted quite often in the corporate world: the CEO who successfully starts a company eventually gets pushed out when the company grows to a certain size. S/he was able to take the company from A to B, but not from B to C. This type of situation offers a rather straightforward reason for replacing a leader, but in other cases an obvious external trigger is not present, and we are forced to look at the deeper psychic elements if we want to glean insight (for example, when a capable leader is pushed out of a group, which is rather common). Even in cases where external forces clearly play a role, the group psyche is of course involved. Our unconscious ability to shape situations to manifest certain outcomes can hardly be overstated.

According to Wilfred Bion (1959), leaders are tolerated for their ability to serve the group towards its goals—conscious or unconscious. Conscious drives may include explicit goals and mission statements. These are the things the group will speak out loud. Amazon.com, for example, states, 'We strive to offer our customers the lowest possible prices, the best available selection, and the utmost convenience'.

Bion (1959) calls this the 'work group'; that part of the group psyche that plans and acts toward the actualisation of explicit value-based tasks.

On the other hand, unconscious drives are not clearly stated but often exert total dominance on the group, and often inhibit completion of the conscious goals. These drives amount to hidden group agendas, such as flight away from a perceived threat. It is common that a group will state one goal and then act in ways that belie a different, unconscious drive. For example, a group that is determined to flee conflict will only authorise leadership that helps the group escape, regardless of any other stated goals.

Bion (1959) asserts that only one group drive is ever active for the group at a given time. While there is only ever one prominent drive at any given moment, the group may switch between drives rather quickly. They tolerate Uranus and his harsh boundaries at first, and then suddenly he is cast aside in favour of Cronus' repressive avoidance (*swallowing the gods*).

Therefore, again, it seems unavoidable that leadership requirements shift as the group stage shifts, and an effective leader avoids assassination by adjusting his/her approach based on these shifts. Effective leaders keep the ultimate values and goals in mind, while balancing the unconscious group drives. They must have a solid compass for the conscious goals of the group while keeping one eye on the unconscious dynamics. This is rare.

More commonly, we see leaders fail to balance the two. One strategy that weak leaders implement is to full-heartedly serve the group psyche's drives at the moment, regardless of the form or direction they take. These leaders may remain in a privileged position in the hierarchy, but this is the death of their own individuality. This type of leader becomes a puppet, and does not lead in any meaningful sense of the word. In extreme circumstances, these are folks who say 'I was only doing my job' in the aftermath of atrocities. We as humans are meant to be more than hollow tools for the group impulses, and fully complying with group impulses means disowning the parts of ourselves that do not fit with the group agenda, so there is a heavy price paid for becoming the group 'yes-man' as a leader.

Idealistic leaders who lack finesse fall on the other end of the spectrum. They fight against group forces, and confront the group from a value-driven, rational stance, but fail to read the deeper drives of the group psyche. In addition to eliciting general resistance from the group, the risk here is that the group may project the persecutor role onto this leader. The line between beloved leader and hated villain is thinner than most realise, and many of the same psychic forces drive the projections behind each. The image of a shaming school teacher losing control of a rowdy classroom comes to mind. Placing oneself as a barrier between the group and its unconscious desires ends poorly.

The wizard apprentice from *Fantasia* loses control of his magic brooms and is washed away in the tide that his creations produce. In post-Jungian thought, this metaphor is especially relevant because, as we will discuss later, water is often thought to symbolise the unconscious. Leaders are often swept away by the powerful rip tide of the group unconscious. In the first example of the complicit leader, they swim with the current willingly out to sea, and in the second example, they thrash wildly the whole time. Either way, underestimating the pull of this current is a deadly sin for a leader.

There is a third mistake that leaders make: The leader could ignore these group forces, which amounts to simply getting out of the way and pretending they do not exist. This type of leader may be tolerated yet estranged from the group. A programme director I knew embodied this strategy. He retained his position, but he lost the respect of colleagues and seemed to become flatter and duller as time passed.

In addition, leadership without the power to shape group outcomes is hollow. These types of leaders become empty figureheads. Worse, this type of leader is ripe for overthrow by a newer voice from the crowd that has explicitly aligned itself to the current unconscious tide. This is different from the 'yes-man' discussed above, in that this role is more passive. The yes-man leader makes a more active alliance with the group's dominant compulsions.

The leader might recognise that many of these options are unfavourable, and it is not uncommon for newer leaders to fantasise about a return to the ranks. Odysseus attempts to flee the call by faking insanity when the Greeks recruit him for the Trojan War.

Odysseus displays another example of cleverness as a leader as well:

> When Odysseus and his men arrive at the island of the Cyclops, they are imprisoned in his cave. The Cyclops, a one-eyed monster born of Poseidon, places a massive boulder blocking the entrance,

which no one can lift but him. In addition to the trapped crew, the monster keeps his sheep in the cave at night, and sleeps there himself. The Cyclops eats a few of Odysseus' crew each day, while the rest watch in powerless horror.

Finally, Odysseus comes up with a plan, and the men take a sharpened stick and stab the Cyclops in his one eye at night while he sleeps, blinding him. He is enraged, but cannot see to attack the men. The next day, as he moves the boulder to let his sheep out one-by-one, he touches the top of each one to ensure that it is a sheep and not one of Odysseus' men trying to escape. Odysseus has his men cling to the underbelly of the sheep, and in this way they are able to escape.

We can associate sheep with the mindless herd mentality. Odysseus rides the belly of the sheep with his men to get through the cave entrance, but then he moves on, boards his ship, and is on his way. He doesn't graze with the sheep or lose himself in the herd, but it is worth noting that 'riding the belly of the sheep' is a technique with which skilled leaders must be familiar. There are times when the wise leader must move gracefully with the salient group compulsions.

While this is sometimes the wise course, masterful leaders need to be able to address group patterns more directly at times too, so that productive movement towards the conscious group goals can occur. This can be as simple as giving a name to what they are observing, since unconscious impulses often lose their power when they are exposed to the light. A leader noticing a scapegoating dynamic might assertively state, 'I'm noticing that we are constantly laying the blame at one person's feet. That's not moving us forward, and we need to think and act like a team', and this can cause a shift in the group. Directness is often warranted, but this process requires finesse. It takes skill to get the toddler to eat the vegetables, and a group psyche often more closely resembles an impulsive toddler rather than a thinking adult. Sometimes a gentler touch can redirect the group momentum just as effectively. That same leader might comment, 'I think there is a place for constructive feedback, but I wonder what we might identify if we focus on our team's strengths?' When facilitators or leaders are not sure of their rapport level with a group, or have evidence that complex dynamics are at play that they do not fully understand, a lighter touch may be a more effective starting point. As a general rule, moving the needle towards more direct, frank, and honest commentary is a good philosophy. Straying from directness tends to be one of the ways facilitators allow the group unconscious to train them to cooperate with the group's own avoidance. If facilitators feel a strong pull to toe around issues, this is data about the system and its patterns.

A skilled leader must surf the group unconscious like a wave, with equal parts attunement, responsiveness, and prediction. Most great leaders do this on an intuitive level, subtly steering the group psyche towards productive means.

Returning to the Odysseus myth, the detail of the boulder may be relevant as well. We know that the Greek gods gave Sisyphus a boulder to push up the hill for eternity as a punishment. Sisyphus' boulder represents a burden, an eternal task. The Cyclops is a terrifying monster, yet he is the one needed to lift the boulder from the entrance and clear the way to escape. Of course, at the same time, he is a terrible threat to the crew. The group unconscious operates in a similar fashion at times. It can be destructive and even 'eat' group members, but it also does some heavy lifting around psychic material that needs resolution or integration. Sometimes we need the monster to lift the boulder.

* * *

We see that the above paints a pessimistic picture for leaders who do not possess skill and maturity, and perhaps even for some that do. This is how it is. Proper leadership is difficult and nuanced and takes time to develop—most leaders fail. The leadership role is desired for the perks, such as a favourable status and access to resources, but there are also risks involved, loneliness to be experienced, and tough choices to be made. Many who ascend to leadership find that the role is not what they expected, and the seduction to avoid real leadership may claim the majority.

Poor leadership is far more common than strong leadership. It would be quite a feat to find an adult with no stories of an incompetent boss. Why do groups recruit incompetent leaders? Or perhaps we should ask why groups mobilise those in leadership to act incompetently.

If we see weak leaders show up so often, we can assume that some part of the group mind wants a weak leader. In other words, when a bad leader is tolerated in a group, it speaks to the group's unconscious desires. For one, weak leadership can reduce the performance expectations placed on us as individuals and for the group-as-a-whole. It may be easier to hold onto fantasies about self-worth when there is little accountability demanded of us to live up to our potential. The group might disguise this type of avoidance by expressing appreciation for a 'relaxed environment'.

Additionally, posting a weak personality in a central leadership role gives groups a ready scapegoating opportunity, and again can provide a buffer between member shortcomings and self-worth. A type of group cohesiveness can even develop among members who can unite in their disdain for the leadership, as discussed previously.

Upper-level leaders may prefer to recruit incompetent mid-level leaders for a similar reason. It can provide a 'meat shield' of sorts; someone to break the bad news and 'discipline the troops', but not receive the glory for crafting the vision. Insecure leaders may also find comfort in knowing their middle management is unlikely to threaten their station with high performance.

Just as incompetent leadership can allow the group to avoid responsibility, an omnipotent saviour as a leader functions in a similar way. What appear to be opposites are perhaps not so far apart after all. In both situations, less may be expected from group members.

When there are active threats to the group's survival in the external environment, a group may be more likely to fantasise about the infallible leader. When the environment is favourable, the group can afford to be less productive, and it may be more likely to recruit an incompetent leader.

When the group recruits a tyrant as a leader, this may signify a group fetish around structure and order. As the old saying goes, Mussolini kept the trains running on time. Group norms may become more crystallised, which can reduce ambiguity and group anxiety. Or perhaps there is a deeper repressed shame that needs to find a channel for expression. We may see groups with shame indulging in a masochistic dynamic, where the leader fulfils the group's fantasy for punishment or atonement of some kind.

In Greek mythology, Uranus was described as a tyrant and harsh father to the Titans. He did not last long. We might consider that a tyrant serves a specific purpose for the group, but may not often allow for long-term equilibrium. If and when the repressed material has been expressed to the group's satisfaction, a Cronus is apt to rise up and sever Uranus' genitals when conditions allow.

If we wish to understand groups, we need to remember that all actions are purposeful, even those that seem to sabotage the group on one level, such as recruiting incompetent or malicious leadership. These benefits exist, but are often well-concealed. Of course, there are also serious costs paid. In addition to the interpersonal unpleasantness and stagnancy we may feel as individual members, incompetent leadership also has sinister effects on the deeper culture of an organisation.

When leadership does fail, what might be the typical outcome, and what relationships are possible between the group and a fallen leader? A common outcome is a death, whether real or symbolic. While literal assassination is an option, exile or social death can often serve to sate the group appetite as well. Dethroned leaders rarely enjoy a powerful role in the system after they are moved out of their leadership role.

Uranus and Cronus leave the mythic narrative entirely once they are dethroned. Set is banished to the Red Sea by Horus as he reclaims the throne in Egyptian lore. An entity which held a strong charge for a leadership role is not simply neutralised. It maintains its charge but reverses polarity, and therefore often experiences a spectacular fall from grace. The group certainly does not say, 'You were the king/queen, so here's 80 per cent of that power in a different position in the new regime'. We rarely see displaced kings return as advisors for their successors. Failed revolts are punished, and overthrown kings are typically disposed of in myth. Ex-leaders carry a strong association with the group drive they served, and as we have discussed, a change in leadership implies a change in salient group drive. This interpretation comes with practical advice for leaders: Don't attempt to reproduce the work of your predecessors, even if you admire them.

The US has a specific system in place to mitigate some of the turmoil that this process typically causes. In the electoral system, we pre-empt the bloody coup by accepting a predictable presidential coup every eight years at the maximum. After two terms, the president is effectively killed off and eliminated from formal leadership. Full-scale overthrows cause large-scale damage. We opt for scheduled, controlled burns in order to reduce the likelihood of massive forest fires. This has drawbacks as well as benefits.

* * *

We discussed previously that leaders are tolerated for their capacity to actualise the current group drives. Sometimes this means that the group demands leaders hold projections for the group, and sometimes this means the leader is tasked to serve as a conduit for connection to certain wanted qualities or attributes, on an archetypical level. This is an important point: leaders can be used by groups in a few different ways, and each has a different feel or quality to it. In the latter situation (leader as connection to archetype), leaders are tolerated to the extent that they can hold the archetype that the group wishes to express. This is a slightly different lens on leadership, similar to Freud's notion of the leader acting as the group's collective ego ideal.

For example, a group manifesting a *fight* drive will likely nomi-nate an Ares or Athena as their leader (formally or informally). There is a real danger here for leaders who get pulled into over-identification with archetypal energies, as is discussed by Edinger in *Eternal Drama* (Edinger, 1994). A type of narcissistic inflation can infect leaders in this position, which typically leads to terrific downfalls. By illustrating the nature and influence of the gods, myth helps to separate the individ-ual from the archetype. Understanding the qualities and content of the archetypes makes it less likely that one will mistake themselves for a god.

Which archetype the group wishes to express (and therefore who is recruited into leadership) depends on the most prominent drive of the group, whether conscious or unconscious. If a leader is not holding a deity for the group—and the right deity, at that—they are apt to be replaced. We might say the group expresses worship of a certain deity or archetype in the leader that it manifests.

Further, when a thing is worshipped, it is likely that it is felt to be missing from the group psyche in some sense. When we project our greatness onto another and declare them to be saviour material, we simultaneously declare ourselves lacking in this quality. The specific longing speaks to what the group believes is missing or needed within the group psyche. In other words, it is not just that the group wishes for a saviour; they need that saviour to have specific qualities that are determined by the context.

Several events in the Trojan War involve the Athenian temples of Troy. Athena, for the most part, supports the Greeks against Troy, so here is evidence that a deity which is felt to be missing is emphasised in worship. It is Athena's idea for the Trojan Horse, after all, which causes the downfall of Troy. The Trojans lacked Athenian support, and the lack of integrated Athena seems to correlate with the compulsion to worship her.

Additionally, worshipping one deity implies a lack of worship for the other archetypes. Just as only one group drive can be centre stage for a group at a given moment, a group cannot properly worship multiple deities simultaneously. The active group drive determines the archetypal longing, so Bion's assertion that only one drive may be active must carry over to the worship symbolism in myth. This is corroborated by the Trojan emphasis on Athenian worship, as her wisdom and warrior prowess were perceived as greatly needed.

Practically speaking, aspiring leaders need to pay attention to the groups' longings, since the group elevates those who serve as vehicles for the archetypes it hopes to express. Stepping into leadership requires holding the right archetype at the right time.

In the leader-as-embodied-archetype situation, leaders' actions make a statement about what behaviours are valued and what behaviours are intolerable. An incapable leader conveys that capability is not valued. A poor communicator in a leadership role signals that healthy communication is not considered a desirable quality by the group. Thus, the neurotic part of the group psyche can recruit a leader lacking in certain qualities to warn and demotivate others from expressing those qualities. It could be that some part of the group psyche feels threatened by those qualities and is actively employing a strategy to repress them. Such artefacts of avoidance hold important information for coaches, consultants, and team leaders hoping to understand their system.

Groups often recruit leaders who struggle to delegate, for example. These types of leaders may be able to do the work themselves, but the skills needed for fruitful collaboration and team planning are missing. When this is the case, we might guess that the group psyche prefers to keep people siloed and separate from each other, and this leader is one of the tools it uses to do so. It belies a distrust towards the forming of productive subgroups. Perhaps there is a subconscious fear among higher leadership of being overthrown. One may recall the Biblical story of the Tower of Babel, in which collaboration among the masses was punished by God, who spread different tongues into the world to sabotage collaboration.

Of course, not all leadership in groups is formalised, and we see informal leaders arise naturally in groups. With informal leaders, the same basic premise holds true: leadership is tolerated to the extent it serves the group's current drive/archetypal longing.

One special type of informal authority exists in the hidden alliances and gossip networks that develop in organisations. These backdoor channels act as an underground grid of power, and the extent of their existence speaks to the level of distrust group members have in the formal leadership to actualise the group drive. If trust in the formal leaders is lacking, gossip and hidden alliances spring up like weeds. Or said differently, if the formal leaders are not addressing the group drives satisfactorily, informal power structures naturally arise. William White (1997) discusses this phenomenon in conflict-ridden workplaces: 'Information about who's doing what to whom becomes an important source of power and self-protection in the organization' (p. 111). Group members will not see this type of activity as a breach of personal integrity if they do not feel that leadership has created a vision with which they are aligned.

Gossip can also help to cement the unwritten values of the group, which is longed for when the formal authority has failed to delineate them in a way that the group psyche can receive. What is often clarified through gossip is, 'Here's what is accepted by the group and what is not'. Clarity of norms is established and individuals can get a better sense of where they stand—at least, this is true for members who are privy to this underground stream of information. Additionally, the act of gossip has the consequence of degrading the relationship between these members and the formal leadership, while simultaneously deepening interpersonal connections between the gossiping members.

There is an agreement made, or a pact signed, between those who engage in destructive gossip. Each knows that the other has done work in the dark, so to speak. Because of distrust in formal authority, individuals prioritise relationships with other specific members over their relationship to the organisation's leadership and stated values. This is what is meant by a hidden alliance.

We discussed the threat of the southern flames, previously—that is to say, the group consuming the individual. Gossip and underground rebellion can also be a way that members defend against this psychic threat. Members can reassert their own individuality and declare differentiation from the group-as-a-whole through the process of gossip. They can maintain connection with one or a few while creating separation from the group-as-a-whole. Doing this in an underground fashion means that they can still experience the benefits of formal group membership.

When a group manifests underground authority, we can ask how this serves the group. The asking of the question is more important than any single correct answer, yet we might start by referencing our previous insight: the group-as-a-whole will not tolerate leadership that does not adequately address (or transmute) the salient group drive. When formal authority fails to align with the group drive, the group recruits underground counter-leadership to get the job done. What formal leadership interprets as sabotage is really just the group unconscious mobilising new leaders towards its goals.

Lastly, there is a hanging question about leadership: Are good leaders always liked? If we measure the quality of leadership by the extent to which a leader helps move a group towards its espoused goals, then the answer is no. Masterful leaders tune in to the unconscious forces of the group, and may exercise some influence on it, but they do not have total control of it. Masterful leaders are better at steering and mitigating the unconscious forces that present obstacles to the espoused goals, and so they are more likely to remain in good standing with the group while being productive.

We certainly should not use popular opinion as a measure of leadership prowess. It says something, but not necessarily the thing we want to know. Popular opinion indicates the extent to which the group psyche feels that the leader is serving the salient group goal. Since the group psyche sometimes selects for harmful short-term goals that threaten healthy long-term goals, sometimes appropriate leadership requires making unpopular decisions. Therefore, we would be wise to be suspicious of leaders who are *always* held in high regard by their group, much as we might be suspicious of a couple that claims to be happy but never has an argument, or a parent that never has conflict with their teen.

It is absolutely possible for the group unconscious to put leaders in a situation in which they must choose between integrity and popularity. To suggest that a good leader, or any leader for that matter, could have complete control of the group unconscious is a fantasy. To hold such a fantasy is to underestimate the power and reach of the group unconscious.

CHAPTER 6

Murder and death

If we can draw meaning from what qualities are tolerated in leadership roles, we can do the same about which qualities are actively extinguished. We can examine death in mythology as a metaphor, and specifically murder. Murder is common in mythic lore, and often creation stories involve murder as a foundational element, as discussed previously.

Whenever a leader is deauthorised or a member's voice is silenced, a murder has taken place. This is overdramatised with intention, of course. The indulgence of the dramatic element makes everything bigger, and bigger things are easier to see.

Murder has a very different tone than a peaceful death. Murder implies a direct action from the group. There is nothing passive about it, even if it is unconscious. Murder implies the presence of strong group motivation to suppress an energy. Group entities or energies are not murdered apathetically; there is a strong feeling involved. This might not appear dramatic in terms of actions taken by the group—they may simply ignore the member to erase them. What we are watching for as facilitators is the emotional charge, the enmity or glee behind the veil.

There is overlap here with the concept of the scapegoat, which we will discuss in more depth later. The scapegoat generally manifests as a single member, subgroup, or external entity which is made to hold multiple unwanted qualities for the group. When we study murderous repression, we are interested in examining a specific flavour of psychic energy that the group is attempting to 'push down', and what that disowning likely implies about the group's unconscious goals.

Our everyday human groups 'murder' members, ideas, and viewpoints with a variety of clever tools: interruptions, changing the topic, cold silence, and outright verbalised hostility. These, of course, are on the more gentle range of the continuum, as human groups are also apt to literal violence and murder.

Yet for such qualities or energies that the group finds disturbing, there are other options besides active repression. In Greek mythology, death generally means relegation to the underworld, but in some cases, spirits are allowed passage to the Blessed Isles or Mount Olympus, which implies a different group process: that of integration. Unsurprisingly, the underworld houses far more spirits than Mount Olympus does.

Regardless of their destination, the elements that are murdered do not ever truly leave the universe (or our group psyche). They go to 'another place', retreating into the recesses of the group psyche (the underworld) until a time when they may again manifest, or ascend to a more conscious level (Mount Olympus). Experienced group therapists or team leaders can corroborate this: cultural or group zeitgeists do not simply disappear. Group patterns remain, even as specific members come and go. This is the magic of culture. If a group has a scapegoat, eliminating the actual scapegoat does not cure the disease of scapegoating. The group will find another vessel to hold the blame, or they will do the necessary work to integrate the psychic material that has been previously repressed. It goes up into the heavens or down into the underworld, but not away.

The myth of Hercules offers us one of these rare upward integrations:

> Hercules is married to Deianeira, but accidentally slays her brother-in-law, and is forced to flee with his wife. At a river crossing, he places Deianeira on the back of the centaur Nessus. During the crossing,

Nessus attempts to violate Deianeira mid-stream, and Hercules shoots him with a poisoned arrow. As Nessus lays dying, he gives some of his blood to Deianeira and tells her it is a love charm and that it can be used to assure Hercules' affection for her. Later, she becomes jealous of Hercules' feelings for Princess Iole, and soaks one of his shirts in the centaur's blood. As he puts on the shirt, he begins to die painfully, for the centaur's blood still carries the poison from Hercules' arrow. He builds a funeral pyre for himself, but as the flames reach his body, he disappears in a flash of lightning and is received by the gods on Mount Olympus.

Hercules stands for strength, but also brutality and rashness, qualities that we often repress. Giving these qualities 'a place in the heavens' is markedly different from pushing them down into the underworld. Integration of such qualities differentiates groups that openly discuss their patterns from groups that deny that any such patterns exist. A group that has integrated brutality might approach member fantasies and dreams of violence with an open curiosity, and without judgement. Groups that integrate shadow material—the unwanted parts—are less prone to impulsively act out such fantasies.

Robert Moore and Douglas Gillette might describe this process as accessing the full archetype through the *axis mundi*. Robert Bly might say that the group has eaten its shadow. Nathaniel Branden might describe this as an expansion of consciousness. Jordan Peterson would say that there is ownership of the inner monster. A group that has integrated its Hercules allows free expression around its strength but also its ugly brutality. After integration, neither is a taboo any more.

The much more common alternative, as discussed, is to push down and repress this energy into the unconscious. This involves a contraction of consciousness. The fantasies, fears, and traits that the group refuses to explicitly own are relegated to the underworld, where they fester and often find ways to resurface at unpredictable places. Fissures open in the Earth, and dark spirits leap up to cause havoc—as Hades rises up to kidnap Persephone, which we will discuss momentarily.

The Greeks give Hercules a place in the sky after his death, but we see many groups shove their Hercules into the underworld. Even in his myth, Hercules visits the underworld briefly in order to fetch Cerberus, the three-headed guardian of the underworld's gate.

It may seem counterintuitive that a group might disown and repress its strength, but this is actually quite common. Mosse and Roberts (in Obholzer & Roberts, 2019) observed this in their work with teams: 'By disavowing power and locating it elsewhere, they reduced their guilt and sense of responsibility, but at the cost of feeling more helpless and vulnerable' (p. 165). We see a repressing of Hercules in groups that come together to vent negatively about work or politics, or groups that seem content to recycle a disempowered narrative of themselves. In these groups it is enormously unpopular to embody power, and members will consciously or unconsciously hide their full talents and capabilities. Victimhood and helplessness become a type of social currency, and weakness is recognised as a virtue. Groups that rally against hierarchy indiscriminately must disown some power. After all, hierarchy is merely the gestalt of power differences. A rigid hierarchy may overemphasise power differences in an unhealthy way, but the destruction of all hierarchy leads to a repression of power itself, which is limiting for the group-as-a-whole and individual members.

And, as we have mentioned, repressed energies find cracks through which they may be expressed, often in an unpredictable and harmful fashion. We recall that Cronus swallowed the gods, yet they burst forth again with a vengeance to be his undoing. The sideways, toxic expression of these energies can also have the effect of reinforcing the group's negative attitude towards the material and cause a redoubling of repressive efforts. Cronus experiences the bottled-up rage of the gods upon their escape, and his fears are validated. Groups that fall victim to the sideways expression of repressed material have their neuroticism reinforced: *I knew that stuff wasn't safe!*

Healthy group norms around assertive communication and authentic feedback can act as deterrents for this type of repression. For this reason, we may see an undermining of safe, open communication as the first assassination committed by a group psyche that is intent upon repression. We might say that in order to effectively push Hercules into the underworld, the group needs to put Apollo there first. Apollo stands for truth and typically spreads awareness to the gods of the happenings on Earth. He is the sun god, and some part of the group psyche intuitively knows that murder is best done in the dark. As we will see in the following myth of Persephone, Helios (the sun personified) is the one to shed light on her abduction by Hades. Shinto mythology offers a case of repression of a sun deity:

> The sun goddess Amaterasu holds dominion over the heavens, and the ocean (or storm) god Susanoo is unsatisfied with his lot and attempts to usurp her throne. He challenges her to a contest to see who can birth more male deities. Susanoo births more, but only by using Amaterasu's possessions to aid him. When she points this out, Susanoo refuses to concede, and instead terrorises her realm, causing Amaterasu to flee to a cave. She remains there while the world languishes without sun, until she hears other gods laughing and ventures out due to curiosity.

It is remarkable in this myth that Susanoo is the god of the ocean, or the storm. Water is often equated with the murky depths of the unconscious by Jungians. Jung (1991) says, 'Water means spirit that has become unconscious' (p. 18). Additionally, we referenced Tuckman's storming phase of groups, in which conflict arises and boundaries are renegotiated. So some force in the unconscious wants to rise up and overthrow the sun. The revealing light of Amaterasu presents a problem for unhealthy group dynamics hoping to be unbottled, so the light of truth is unseated as a first order of business. We experience this when dealing with those who attack logic and reason themselves. If rational thought is allowed to be marginalised as a tool of a corrupt system, the sun is put into the cave. Some would argue that in the US the erosion of trust in the news media amounts to a killing off of Amaterasu, or Apollo, or Helios.

I brought this myth up—and my associations—to an old mentor of mine during the 2020 riots in the US. He claimed that his political party was trying to 'break the sun goddess out'. Yet it is curiosity that brings out Amaterasu, not aggression. Curiosity becomes a bold stance in the presence of repressive forces. Veteran organisational consultant and group relations practitioner James Krantz says that curiosity is the cure for projection. When it is taboo to ask honest questions, we can be sure that the sun is in the cave, and our group is stuck in a trance of sorts. Of course, genuine curiosity needs to be differentiated from preconceived, agenda-laced lines of questioning.

In repressive groups, the first unwritten rule is that the patterns are not to be discussed. These types of groups react with hostility to those who attempt to bring awareness to the dynamic, and this is good information for any would-be leader to keep in mind. A group need is being met through its behaviour, and shining a light haphazardly on the dynamic is often experienced by the group as threatening. It should only be done with intentionality, following some serious thought about what the repressive dynamic may be accomplishing for the group psyche.

Persephone, the goddess of spring and nature, is not murdered *per se*, but she is abducted to the underworld by Hades, which we can interpret in a similar light:

> Persephone, the adored daughter of the goddess Demeter, is strikingly beautiful and desired by Hades. One day, while picking flowers, she wanders away from her companions to pick the beautiful Narcissus bloom. As she bends down to pick the flower, the ground opens up and Hades appears and abducts her to the underworld to be his queen. Demeter searches for Persephone for nine days until she finds Helios, the sun, who gives her an account of Persephone's abduction. Demeter finds that Zeus had known about the kidnapping and had given permission, and is so angered that she leaves Olympus. She places a curse on the Earth that causes plants to wither.
>
> Zeus becomes worried as the Earth becomes more and more desolate, and eventually sends Hermes down to fetch Persephone back from the underworld. However, Persephone eats some pomegranate seeds from the underworld, which seals Hades' claim to her. She is allowed to live on the Earth for eight months of the year, but must return to the underworld for the remaining four. When Persephone returns to the underworld each year, the Earth experiences winter, and nothing grows.

Again, we see that material which is pushed down in the psyche tends to resurface again. In this case, Persephone returns to the surface world as the herald of springtime. Persephone represents rejuvenative forces, another set of qualities that we might not expect groups to disown at first glance. Yet, as we observed with Hercules, groups may repress parts of themselves that might normally be thought of as positive, depending on circumstances and the salient narrative. Traditionally toxic masculine groups, such as some football locker rooms or college fraternities, push Persephone into the underworld. Any groups that are intolerant of vulnerability among members encourage her abduction. In a cultural context lacking in emotional (or physical) safety, the ability to protect oneself takes centre stage. Survival depends on maintaining an image of toughness, physically and/or emotionally. Expressing Persephone energy is likely to get one taken advantage of in this context.

In such groups, which may range from cut-throat law firms to inner-city gangs, Hercules walks around proudly and Persephone is pushed into the underworld. In any group where vulnerable generativity is not celebrated, the deal is made with Hades to rise up and snatch Persephone away.

None of this is to say that Persephone or Hercules should be fully expressed at all times in order for a group to be considered healthy. It is more of a question of where these energies are placed within the group psyche. A group of soldiers in the middle of a firefight needs to channel Hercules, not Persephone. But when either is a taboo, and the group remains unable to access the energies when appropriate, something important is lost.

Of stories involving murder, the theme of revenge is common—indeed, we see threads of it in both examples above. Vengeance may move up the power ladder, such as in the Babylonian tale of Gimil-Ninurta, wherein a pauper seeks violent retribution against the mayor of his city. Likewise, in the Inca creation myth, one of the first men, Wichama, avenges his mother's death at the hands of the creator god Pacha Kamaq, driving the god into the sea. Yet, we also see examples of more powerful figures seeking revenge on those in less powerful stations. The Greek goddesses Athena and Hera vow to destroy the city of Troy as retribution against Paris for choosing Aphrodite as the fairest goddess. In the Epic of Gilgamesh, the goddess Ishtar seeks revenge against the mortal Enkidu after his threatening words, and kills him with a prolonged illness. Those in power are capable of feeling wronged by those in less powerful positions. Indeed, it has been my experience that leaders often feel underappreciated or wronged by their team. This often comes as a surprise to members.

The Greeks give us Nemesis, the goddess of retribution. Nemesis is said to be the daughter of Nyx, the goddess of night, and to have no father. It seems strange from our lens of modernity that the archetypal goddess of vengeance is not only female, but even lacks the masculine element of a father. One might expect a masculine association, given the aggression implied in revenge, and the typical connection the literature makes between masculinity and aggression, but this is not the case. The drive for retribution originates with the perception of being wronged. Without such a wound, there does not arise the drive for revenge. As we will discuss later, we do get some sense that the feminine in our culture has received systemic wounding, and we have mobilised the feminine to seek a rebalancing with certain masculine elements within society through movements such as 'Time's Up'.

Mythic revenge involves repressed group psychic material rising back up 'with a vengeance'. It is the direct storytelling of the theme we have touched on: that which is pushed down finds a way to rise back to the surface.

Working with this group material can be challenging as a leader. In my experience, it helps to set aside specific times in the work week to explore the potential taboos of the group culture. You can do this using a journal, your team, or an external coach. The presence of taboos implies the sun goddess is stuck in the cave. And as we recall, putting her there is a likely prerequisite to the murderous group drives being acted out. Recognition of this is an important first step. Then, we can start to disarm and pre-empt these drives by skilfully opening up dialogue.

A leader needs to gauge the temperature of repressive energies, and find a reasonable starting point to get curious with their team. It is important to recognise when bringing in an outside facilitator may be beneficial; the best thing a leader can often do is to approach such volatile energy with a sense of humility. A good rule of thumb is that if you as a leader feel an emotional charge around a dynamic, consider a different entry point for dialogue (and do your own emotional work around that dynamic).

Cancel culture: A modern application

Aodhán Moran

The phrase 'cancel culture' has become a popular way to describe coordinated attacks on figures for perceived offences. Within cancel culture, individuals deemed to have acted unacceptably are publicly shamed, stripped of accolades, and ostracised. In what can be seen as a collective defence mechanism, fears, insecurities, and flaws are put into cancelled individuals, who then become a *persona non grata*. Like Hitler triggering a disgust response by labelling Jews vermin, cancelled individuals become contaminated in the collective imagination.

Often comedians, whose archetypal role as Jester necessitates political incorrectness, have their jokes used against them by the crowd. There are many examples of content producers deceptively editing snippets from long-form interviews out of context, in such a way that the interviewees' intended message is twisted into something that sounds wildly combative, and clearly diverges from the interviewee's original intentions. What is the motivation for this, from a psychological perspective? Remember our golden rule of projection: what is most condemned is often repressed or not integrated.

Dr Simon Western put forward that the political correctness (PC) associated with cancel culture stems from a place of emotional wounding: anything that can be viewed as hateful towards marginalised groups—gays, women, or racial minorities—activates the personal 'wounded self'. Out of this pain, the 'PC tribe' are driven to protect the weak from these painful experiences. Heightened sensitivity and compassion are characteristic traits of the PC tribe. Repression of less-PC traits such as aggression and hostility is encouraged. As with all repressed energy, it does not go away, and in some cases it manifests as intense passive aggression. Subtle attacks on hierarchy and power can be funnelled through the veil of compassion for those on the margins. This is Thanatos (the drive toward death and destruction) shrouded in Eros (the drive toward life and love).

Some of these cancel culture tendencies emerged during an intergroup event at a residential group relations conference I attended.

The conference membership was racially and ethnically diverse, with members coming from Australia, Belgium, Brazil, China, Colombia, Jamaica, Denmark, Finland, India, Ireland, Israel, Italy, Norway, Palestine, South Africa, Turkey, the Netherlands, the United Kingdom, and the United States. While we had the English language as a common denominator, the diversity created a space rife with the potential for miscommunication and misunderstanding.

The primary task of this event was to study the relationship and relatedness of members and staff in the here and now, bringing into focus authority and authorisation. Because this intergroup event took place about halfway through the conference, the membership had already participated in many sessions together, giving time for relational patterns to emerge.

At the beginning of the conference, an individual in the membership, who we will refer to as X, felt that they had been racially mislabelled by the conference director. On another occasion, X brought ethnic food from outside the conference to share with the membership, only to have it confiscated and thrown out by venue management, who feared that potential food poisoning would be associated with the food on their property. Recalling the links between disgust response and cancel culture, poisoning and disgust are tightly linked, inciting powerful negative affect.

Later, X participated in a subgroup of younger, ethnically diverse members in leading a premeditated subversion of the large group. When someone outside their circle spoke, they stood; when it was silent, they remained seated. Their explicit intention was to emphasise the need for silence and to rebel against the elders for deauthorising them. Like Zeus overthrowing Cronus, the large group rebellion suggested disenchantment with the current hierarchy, and a desire to form their own.

In a space where something as simple as checking the time has meaning, a premeditated attack on the formal structure brings with it many questions. Following the premise that nothing in this work is a coincidence, we might ask what in the group psyche was mobilising these individuals to rebel. How was this experienced by the elders? For the rebels themselves? For the consultants?

One of the elders responded aggressively by loudly chastising the rebels for wasting the members' time and, and after some back and forth, left the room. Reflecting on this, I empathised with the elder, but at the time, I lacked the awareness and courage needed to go against the rebels. When questioned later as to why I did not join the rebels, I replied that 'I wished I was as brave as them'. Looking back on the situation, I was veiling Thanatos with Eros. I was stuck between two opposing energies: on one hand, wanting to please everybody; on the other, defending against feelings of disgust and contempt. In the end I withdrew in meek silence.

Unchallenged by peers, X's group eventually began acting as an informal management team, directly challenging the formal leaders of the conference. They commandeered conference rooms and put out formal invitations for other subgroups to disregard the instructions of management. X had been primed to become a voice for the perceived victims, and the group psyche was using them as a vehicle to cancel the explicit authority and attack the hierarchy.

These dynamics came to a head during the aforementioned intergroup event. During this section of the conference, X's group commandeered a room that had been intended for part of the staff team. Rather than using the space designated by conference staff to interface with other groups, they invited all other groups, including management, to a room of their choosing. X's group attempted to take control of the event by changing the focus of the primary task from the *relationship between membership and staff* to the *relationship between groups*. X's group also took notes of what management said and then read them aloud to the membership.

Here we see inklings of what Howard Schwartz called the maternal matrix and the loss of the symbolic Father (Schwartz, 1997, as cited by Western, 2017). The collective imagination sees only the negative aspect of the Father (Tyrant Beast), dismissing the positive aspect (Wise King). All the qualities associated with the Father—tradition, boundaries, authority—are viewed as structures of oppression. In cancel culture, there is no room for nuance: the Father, authority, and hierarchy are evil and should be metaphorically (and sometimes literally) *murdered*. Schwartz asserts that PC culture is a bid for power in the name of the Primitive Mother, expelling the Father, and undermining the paternal function. The problem here is that killing the symbolic Father is also killing his benevolent aspects: boundaries, culture, organisation, and socialisation.

Within any group setting, a cancel culture creates an environment where free speech is not possible. Unable to communicate openly, for fear of being ostracised, group members begin to walk on eggshells. As a result, the group's capacity for real thinking is diminished. As soon as something is inevitable, no learning can emerge. This means that the hardest conversations may also offer the greatest productive movement for groups, especially in therapeutic or learning settings.

CHAPTER 7

Unions and pairings

Murder is one type of interaction in myth, but there are of course others. The ancient stories are rife with character unions—both romances and rivalries. Wilfred Bion highlights group tendencies to pair specific members together, as a union of sorts. From a group-as-a-whole perspective, we say that unions occur when the group colludes to bring two members together to accomplish something for the group on a psychic level. In myth, this means that there is a story to tell involving two characters and what they represent, and the same can be said for our everyday groups. We can think of each member involved as holding specific archetypal energy, and these can give us clues about what the unconscious is 'up to'.

Pairings evoke emotion from the group, as opposed to indifference. This is one of the ways we can recognise a true pairing. We as group members are instruments; if we feel deeply one way or another when two specific members interact, this is evidence of pairing. The group will likely focus keenly on the chosen pair's interactions, whereas other members may be interrupted or ignored. Romance between members is an obvious way pairing manifests, yet sometimes it looks like a conflict between two members that the group cannot seem to escape.

If the group consistently returns to a conflict or specific connection between certain members, we can conclude there is some sort of pairing attraction present. Bion might have argued that unions born of conflict indicate a different group process; We are suggesting that often a dyad pulled into constant conflict is actually a type of pairing.

Why would a group desire to bring two energies together at all? Bion hypothesised that pairings within a group reveal the subconscious longing for a saviour to be born from the union. When a beautiful couple pairs in real life, people cannot help themselves: they will imagine what kind of baby the couple might produce. The specific individuals, and what they stand for, can speak to the qualities that the group desires in their saviour.

In more broad and applicable terms, we can hypothesise that groups pair specific members together in service of meeting group goals (which are often unconscious)—to produce *something* or perhaps ameliorate an undesirable internal state. A group may recruit two attractive members to flirt while the rest watch, to escape a brewing conflict with outside forces. Or the group may feel stuck in grief after a beloved member departs, and pull in an emotional member and a nurturing member to help act out the grieving process. Something is desired, and the group is mobilising internal members as resources in order to achieve it.

Dr Simon Western teaches the Lacanian idea that desire arises from lack. If a group longs for a thing, it follows that it does not currently possess the thing. The longing implies that the desired qualities are absent in an integrated form from the group consciousness. Each union is an attempt at alchemy. The group brings two elements together in hopes of producing the missing ingredient that will deliver the group into a higher state or resolve painful emotions. Because of this, unions can inform our approach to membership or leadership in groups.

Myths leave us with another clue. Since myths follow a story format, they do not merely give us information about what gets paired. They also give us clues about the likely outcomes of specific pairings. We can use mythological pairings and their progeny to make predictions about the outcome of such attempted alchemy in our everyday groups. Additionally, we can view successful mythical unions as a blueprint for successful integration of qualities in groups. Ares (war) and Harmonia (harmony) come together and give birth to the Amazons, the female warrior race that has an important place in the Greek stories. Our modern culture resists the idea that aggression and harmony have a place together, so it should be no surprise that the Western world is still searching for an honoured place to put its integrated feminine Warrior.

Many mythological entities are associated with multiple traits, and so divining which traits are salient in a given pairing can be a murky endeavour. We have the Egyptian pairing of Isis and Osiris. Isis represents healing and magic (Britannica, 2024), while Osiris represents fertility, agriculture, the dead, resurrection, and life (Frazer, 1922). Which of these might be relevant? There is no objective measuring stick. An interpretation is successful if it increases the depth of questions we ask about the groups we wish to understand, or raises our awareness of discrepancies between our groups and the myths. This does not imply we should be striving to act in accordance with myths, *per se*, but awareness of group rejection of archetypes is helpful.

We should note that Osiris and Isis are both siblings and a couple. We will discuss mythic incest in more depth in the next chapter, but for now we can say that incest involves pairing two similar energies within a group. Indeed, we see shared symbols between Osiris and Isis involving life and regeneration.

In the myth, Osiris' evil brother Set betrays him and locks him in a chest, then eventually chops him into fourteen pieces. Isis recovers thirteen of the pieces and revives Osiris, but his genitals are eaten by fish. We have the castrated masculine, repaired by the divine healing feminine.

We could construe this myth as a parable of group rejection of homogenous leadership. Osiris and Isis were siblings and overlapped in their representations. A dark force within the group rises up and tears down the inbred leadership.

The malicious Set energy within a group is good for an overthrow, but cannot sustain a thriving kingdom. This is common for real-life groups. Hidden alliances and toxic gossip that serve to undermine a leader or authority do not nourish the group once the leader is gone. What has been broken up and scattered must be repaired and integrated again before a healthier world order can be established.

Yet the union of Osiris and Isis also brings a son named Horus, the falcon-headed god of kingship and the sky. Horus acts as the balance-restorer, bringing prosperity back to the land and driving Set into the Red Sea. So there is some ambivalence present; the homogenous pairing is overthrown but also produces a saviour. Our culture reflects this ambivalence towards incest, or like-with-like pairings. Increasing diversity has become part of the stated agenda for corporations, yet at the same time the public supports an entire genre of incestual erotic fiction novels.

Of course, not all unions happen between masculine and feminine energies. In the Babylonian Epic of Gilgamesh, we see a male–male pairing as an important part of the story arc:

> Gilgamesh, a Sumerian king, is known as a tyrant and feared by his people. He is lust-driven and abducts women at will from among his subjects. His people pray to the fertility goddess Aruru to fashion a man who can overpower Gilgamesh, so that the women of the city can be left in peace. Aruru creates the mighty Enkidu, a hairy man with bull's legs who lives out with the wild beasts.
>
> Upon hearing about the Wild Man, Gilgamesh sends a courtesan to seduce Enkidu, and after Enkidu lies with her, his animal friends no longer associate with him. Upon losing his connection to his animal friends, he follows the courtesan back to the city of Uruk.
>
> In the palace, Gilgamesh dreams of struggling with a powerful man who can master him. Gilgamesh's mother interprets the dream to mean that he and Enkidu will become great friends. And indeed, after a hard-fought wrestling match, Enkidu and Gilgamesh become as brothers.
>
> In later adventures, we see a noble side of Gilgamesh emerge, as he goes to great lengths in an attempt to bring immortality to his people.

Here we have the abusive masculine power paired with the innocent Wild Man energy. The immature masculine energy—what Moore and Gillette (1992) called the Tyrant archetype—is running rampant in the group, and the feminine element is being disregarded and violated. The story implies that Wild Man energy within the group is what is required to regulate the tyrant. The longing of the group behind this pairing is hinted at: appropriate balance and regard for the feminine.

There is feminine energy actively involved in the story as well, as it is a goddess who releases the Wild Man into the world, and a female courtesan who seduces Enkidu and brings him to the city. The birth and evolution of the Wild Man requires aid from the feminine. Male wildness is not contrary to femininity, it is connected to it. Fertility and earthliness go hand in hand with the Wild Man. On the other hand, the toxic masculine lives in the city centre, and experiences women as sexual objects, or subjects to be sent on errands. Gilgamesh does not have a deep relationship with the natural world. He sends a courtesan to interact with the natural world on his behalf. The myth validates our suspicion of the powerful men in our culture who do not take steps to stay connected with nature. Men who wear fancy suits on weekdays and avoid spending time in the wild are stuck channelling this undeveloped iteration of Gilgamesh.

Additionally, the myth implies that the Tyrant is not integrated by shaming or manipulation. There is a boldness in the confrontation between Enkidu and Gilgamesh. Through the wrestling match, Enkidu meets Gilgamesh with a language he can understand, and this is what is required for the evolution of Gilgamesh from Tyrant to virtuous King.

The detail about the dream is potent. The Tyrant has a dream (or fantasy) of being dominated, or 'mastered', by the Wild Man. There may be a sexual connotation here, implying that the abusive masculine is ultimately driven by longing for domination itself. But we find more meaning in a less provocative perspective: The uninitiated masculine longs for integration with the healthy Wild Man and perhaps the experience of something bigger than itself. It wants to experience containment and limits.

Applying the group-as-a-whole framework, we can say that the effective handling of toxic patriarchy involves a union with the healthy Wild Man. Men need to reclaim the healthy wildness, and feminine energy is involved in this process. The unhealthy patriarchy needs to be confronted from male strength, and with the hope of evolving perspectives, as opposed to shaming and condemning Gilgamesh. After all, after his union with Enkidu, Gilgamesh goes on to endure great sacrifice for his people.

Our cultural response to Gilgamesh is not in line with the myth, and perhaps as a result, we are not experiencing our Gilgamesh transform from a Tyrant into a King archetype. One side of the aisle seems intent on burning down Gilgamesh's castle with torches, holding 'Time's Up' banners, and in response we see the abusive male energies digging in their heels and doing what they do best: preparing for battle. While anger (and defensiveness) can be understood, something gets lost here. Trauma sets in deeper when we strip Gilgamesh of his humanity. It violates our group-as-a-whole understanding to try and shove our collective toxic patriarchy down into the dirt. The shadow must be integrated for the healing to occur.

Additionally, the feeling on the street is that masculine strength belongs only to the Gilgameshes among us, and this is an unhelpful perspective in many ways. Masculine power should not be conflated with abusive masculine power, or else we write off Enkidu. This amounts to Enkidu staying out in the wild, unseen. Our story hints that the Wild Man strength needs to be seen or touched by some feminine element before it 'comes to the city'.

So we can take something away from the Babylonian epic about how to deal with warped masculinity. This pairing offers a potential prescription for the fractured masculine, a condition which plagues our society currently at great cost. Perhaps we can take solace in the fact that we have myths that seem to speak to this condition and potentially hint at paths towards archetypal healing.

CHAPTER 8

Incest and group diversity

Among unions, incest appears as a special subcategory that can provide clues to understanding group attitudes on diversity. We see sibling unions in Greek literature with Uranus and Gaia, Cronus and Rhea, and Zeus and Hera, among others. In Egyptian myth, Isis and Osiris are paired, along with other siblings such as Shu and Tefnut. Incestual unions by definition offer very little diversity; they are pairings marked by sameness.

King Arthur's myth provides us with such a pairing:

> As King Arthur rises to power, many noblemen, knights, and ladies visit his court. Among these is the noblewoman Morgause. Morgause falls in love with Arthur and they conceive a child together, Mordred. After the encounter, Arthur discovers that he shares a parent with Morgause, and thus he has slept and conceived a child with his own half-sister. Mordred, the child, grows up to be an evil knight and brings destruction to Arthur's court.

Let us again assume that myth provides a mirror for our group psyche, and therefore that groups on some level feel a pull towards pairing entities with similarities.

While not a ubiquitous theme in world myths, there are examples of incest in the early stages of myths producing powerful disruptors or conquerors. Mordred is one such example, and we might also point to Uranus and Gaia birthing Cronus (who dethrones Uranus), or Cronus and Rhea birthing Zeus (who dethrones Cronus).

This fits nicely with organisational psychology and observations about diversity. The value of diversity to a group depends largely on the task of the group and the current stage of group development, according to the work of Gunter Stahl's team at Vienna University (2010). For example, during brainstorming tasks early in a project, teams are served well by having access to variegated perspectives. Any task that is complicated may benefit from diversity of thought. Idea incest in these situations is severely limiting for groups.

On the other hand, when a group or team enters a phase of executing a strategy or the task is simple and straightforward, too many different perspectives can lead to disarray. At times when the troops need to be in lockstep, diversity causes more harm than good. In these instances, the proverbial incest can be appropriate. There is a benefit in pairing like with like when the task is crystallised and linear.

Groups tend to be suspicious of differences among members. However, in my experiences with group work, it is not all differences that mobilise suspicion and biases of group members. Differences and similarities become salient when they have relevance towards the primary group goal of the moment, whether the goal is conscious or not. Member differences that are perceived to move a group closer to the goal are likely to be tolerated or celebrated. When the member differences are seen as a hindrance to the group goal (or when a fight is the unconscious group goal), toxic highlighting of these differences is likely to occur. The group may fracture in some sense, splitting off subgroups to hold different parts of itself in a manner that allows some members to disown the troubling qualities, as discussed previously.

Race relations is a perennial hot topic and can be viewed through this lens. Race is certainly not always a divisive factor in racially diverse groups, but tends to be a ready vehicle for group attitudes around member differences to surface.

Just as some groups may deny the impact of the racial history on current social dynamics, other groups may tend to overemphasise it or latch on to distorted projections. If the White man is made to hold the blame as persecutors, then other subgroups may feel a psychic burden lifted, or a freedom from certain responsibilities. The problem becomes systemic racism on the part of White people and any question of other cultural factors is disregarded. The trap exists in reverse as well. Black men have been made to hold the projection of violent criminal activity. Of course, both of these common responses involve projection in an unhealthy way. Biases exist and affect minorities and all subgroups, and also, there is a possibility of the group-as-a-whole 'taking back' projections.

One should be suspicious of anyone who claims the issue is simple or linear. That is to say, humility and curiosity are the appropriate tools to bring to the table if we are hoping to build bridges instead of burn them, regardless of our own skin colour, ethnicity, or membership in a subgroup.

As mentioned in our last chapter, race discussions tend to produce strong emotional responses, so it is helpful to remember that group-as-a-whole work demands an investigative and open stance towards the deeper group psyche. Again, it is curiosity that brings the sun goddess Amaterasu out of her cave.

Likewise, it would be unhelpful to conclude that group biases against minorities (or majorities) are purely toxic and reflect character flaws on the part of individual members. This implies a lack of understanding of group dynamics. It is not simply that people and groups are stupid or evil. Ultimately, these biases have roots as a protective mechanism for the groups and individuals, as discussed above. After all, the Trojans accepted a 'gift from the other' when they took in the Trojan Horse unexamined, and it caused their city's ruin. Suspicion acts as a group defence. We can work with biases and stereotypes better when we seek to understand how they are serving the group.

We have a bind, because when these biases are activated they inhibit opportunities for minority members, which clearly violates many of our ideas about fairness and equality. Yet these defences have served human groups in the past and relate to unconscious group drives that we cannot eliminate by shaming. There is not an easy fix here, but increasing understanding of group dynamics is a preferred strategy over shaming the group resistance to minority membership/leadership and simply forcing it into place. This typically does not end with positive results.

Just as repressed material resurfaces, energies that are elevated without proper support will tend to crash back down to earth again. Putting a minority member into a leadership role in a group without providing systemic support and resolving resistance is setting this person up for failure, which then reinforces negative biases towards that minority group. A more skilled approach involves two tactics.

First, group resistance needs to be recognised as a survival mechanism, as opposed to evilness. Suspicion of novelty and difference has increased the odds of survival in our evolutionary past. Leaders are more likely to increase openness to diversity by accepting the positive intent behind the defence mechanism, as opposed to shaming it. Shaming tends to entrench viewpoints.

Bill Plotkin and Thomas Berry (2003) use the metaphor of the loyal soldier to express this idea: When Japan surrendered in World War II, they left stranded soldiers on Pacific islands with no way to communicate to them that the war was over. These soldiers maintained a fanatic loyalty to their cause and a hostile orientation towards strangers. These were considered virtuous attributes during the war, but problematic during peacetime. It was found that the best response to these soldiers was to honour them for their service, rather than attempt to argue them into cooperation. Our group defence mechanisms, like the loyal soldiers, exist in our group psyche for a reason, and we will get farther towards disarming them by honouring the ways they have served us.

Second, a leader or group facilitator must find opportunities to emphasise the salient similarities between minority members and the group-as-a-whole. The narrative around sameness is important here, rather than any objective truth. After all, no human is the same as any other, and every group member will be a minority in some way. Skilled navigators find ways to emphasise the important similarities that have a positive bearing on group goals (again, conscious or unconscious). This is a necessary ingredient for camaraderie. At a basic level, a leader needs to convey the message to subordinates that 'We are alike in some ways that are important'. This decreases the distance that the group psyche needs to travel in terms of accepting difference. Some leaders instinctively do this in a toxic way, through the creation of an external (or internal) enemy that allows the group to rally together and identify with each other in the common cause. Healthy groups do it without scapegoating.

Of course, in any group, the cultural biases of the individuals are part of the soil in which the group dynamics take root. This being said, from the group-as-a-whole lens, we are particularly curious about how groups mobilise these biases. The question is not whether discriminatory judgement is present. We might instead ask:

- Which member differences seem to be emphasised?
- How might the emphasis on these differences be serving the group-as-a-whole?
- How can we highlight shared valuable attributes of members?

CHAPTER 9

Attraction and contempt

A ttraction between members is certainly a factor in pairings, but it is also a bigger concept in its own right.

In group relations work, attraction tends to be one of the most thrilling, taboo, and potentially dangerous topics that emerge. Questions around who is authorised to express and receive attraction, and who is 'left out in the cold' become relevant and give us clues about the group. Attractions between members may become a vehicle towards undermining boundaries, both on the individual level or on a group level.

One *Merriam-Webster* definition for *lust* is 'an intense longing'. It is the opposite of measured, conscious energy. Lust has a manic energy to it; the flame burns hot. The objects of a group's lust reveal much about the underlying group drives. We recall that Dr Simon Western takes a Lacanian perspective on desire and encourages us to look at lust as a signifier of a felt lack. Following Western's thinking, desire in groups indicates some unmet need, and we as facilitators can opt to take a curious stance. That which is lusted after becomes a clue towards understanding the group psyche.

In normal parlance, lust typically refers to a strong positive attraction. Yet, groups also paradoxically find themselves *lustful of conflict*, too.

The Norse phrase *bloodlust* becomes relevant, or the idea of seeing red (red being the colour of passion, according to Robert Bly and Robert Johnson).

As is a theme in this work, we take the stance that opposites may be more closely related than previously thought. Both hatred and deep attraction move us out of rational thought and into the realm of the unconscious. As we discussed previously, a hated enemy often provides value to the group as an external target at which to direct unified malice. They are an outlet for psychic material that is too hot to handle internally. Likewise, objects of group lust serve some unconscious purpose for the group.

The Lumineers write, 'The opposite of love (is) indifference', implying that it is helpful to imagine lust and animosity not as opposites but as closely related in terms of the emotional charge that each carries. The line between contempt and positive attraction can be thinner than we realise. It may be more useful to think of these as two poles of a magnet. The north and south poles of a magnet are opposites but also closely related. They are reliant on the presence and potential of the other—and additionally, magnetic poles can be reversed. Often in group relations work, uttering the word 'attraction' shifts the energy from passionate death (Thanatos) to passionate love (Eros) in an instant.

This is an important principle: Attraction can underpin conflict in groups. This is not so far away from the mechanics behind a schoolboy acting nasty towards a girl on whom he has a crush. It is a cry for intimacy and attention. As facilitators, if we can avoid taking conflicts at face value and instead explore potential attraction, oftentimes we can generate helpful insight into how a particular group system is operating.

Thanatos to Eros

Aodhán Moran

These types of dynamics come to life quickly in group relations conferences, where members are tasked to examine the patterns they encounter in the here and now with their assigned groups.

In one conference, within a small group that had experienced some relational discord, a member (we will call her 'B') shared a dream she had: Walking around a village in the dead of night, she broke into houses and systematically murdered sleeping occupants. In her dream, she enjoyed this streak of violence, which was a complete departure from her typical persona.

Immediately after B's contribution, words of aggression and violence circulated the group, punctuated by long, pregnant silences. Self-expression in any vulnerable sense felt dangerous.

That said, themes of murder and violence were not resonating with me. When spoken words have no emotional resonance, when they feel empty, it is worth considering their authenticity. Are they covering something deeper?

Just when things felt as if they would boil over, our group consultant provided an intervention: 'Sure, blood is associated with murder and death, but it also is associated with new life, with birth'. Following the consultant's intervention, I acknowledged my attraction toward a member of the group. The conversation tiptoed from words of murder to words of passion. B openly wondered if the passionate murder they were circling around was really a cover for passionate love. B's dream moved the group psyche toward Thanatos, while the consultant's intervention shed light on Eros.

Also, both positive attraction and deep hostility towards an entity can begin to shape the identity of a group. There are times when it becomes hard to imagine what a group's identity would be if a specific conflict were to disappear. Freud might comment that the external entity in these cases, whether loved or hated, has been introjected into the group ego (Freud, 1921b).

In the US, much of the liberal identity consists of opposition to Trump, and the same may be said of conservatives towards certain mainstream media outlets like CNN. We can say that there is a strange dependence or lust involved. It has the feel of addiction for both sides. The right uses China, the left uses Russia, and both parties use each other to ground their own identity. There is security when there is something dependable to push against.

The Trojan War mixes conflict and attraction from the outset. It begins with a competition between the goddesses Hera, Athena, and Aphrodite for the title of fairest.

> Discord tosses a golden apple into the assembly of gods on Olympus, and the apple is marked with the words 'for the fairest'. Aphrodite, Hera, and Athena all make a claim, and cannot come to an agreement. Paris, a prince-turned-shepherd, is chosen to judge the contest and give the golden apple to the winner. He chooses Aphrodite, who promises him the hand of the beautiful Helen as a bride if she wins. His choice angers both Athena and Hera, who vow to destroy him and all of Troy.

Aphrodite, representing lust, outcompetes Athena (goddess of wisdom) and Hera (goddess of marriage, among other things) to win the golden apple from Paris. Wisdom and stable relationships take a backseat to lust. This feels familiar to our modern perspective. Culturally, we choose Aphrodite, yet become indignant when we endure our own Trojan War. We give the golden apple to *Jersey Shore* and Kim Kardashian, so we should not be surprised by exploitative media, corrupt politics, declining schools, and deteriorating personal relationships.

In our boardrooms, we like to pretend that Aphrodite does not hold our apple. The fantasy exists that we are guided by Athena in her wisdom or Hera in her integrity. Lust and attraction are strong drivers of group behaviour that are almost always pushed down into the basement of the group psyche in organisational contexts. The tendency in academic and business teams is to downplay the sexuality of members. In professional (and most non-professional) settings, it is seen as uncouth to discuss group dynamics at a sexual level in the here and now. William White (1997) points out in *The Incestuous Workplace* that, except for sexual harassment, there is a conspicuous dearth of literature on sexuality as an organisational dynamic (p. 96). Lust is rarely discussed in the open, even though the attractions that occur in groups are a large part of the excitement that comes with grouping. It is the norm that we set aside Athena and Hera to experience Aphrodite as a group, as our story suggests. Preserving the taboo quality of acknowledging it seems to be a part of the enjoyment.

This is not to say that groups should force the subject. There is clearly wisdom in avoiding the topic when group goals would be jeopardised by tensions that might result. Yet, it is helpful to remember this if we are working with a team that claims total openness in communication.

The lack of discussion around attraction reveals that this is a fantastical narrative, and potentially part of an elaborate architecture of avoidance parading as openness.

Attraction often correlates with perceived physical beauty, but there are myriads of other factors that intertwine to determine the attractive pull of individual members. In one small group during a conference, I observed the men develop a strong attraction for a middle-aged pregnant woman (in the presence of several younger women who would typically be considered attractive). In another instance, a strong connection formed between a gay man and a straight man, causing envy among some of the straight women. The common theme is that these members exuded some type of pull, or power.

Attraction and power are often closely related. Power is a dirty word in our culture currently, but it is also one of the primary factors underlying attraction. This doesn't just mean formal power, although groups will often hold an attraction (or repulsion) towards members in formal power. Physical beauty—and the implied reproductive capability—is power, a strong intellect is power, capability with one's hands is power, and the ability to create fun is power. Power is the ability to move towards productive ends, which means that it is a moving target, since group goals change over time. Experiencing a sense of power is also a basic group need, as it implies the capacity to move towards the goals—conscious or unconscious—of the group. Members who exhibit power related to the salient group goals in the moment are likely to be seen as attractive.

The group unconscious elevates certain traits as attractive in connection with its goals, which come with expectations. Some members may invite and even abuse this power. Others may become uncomfortable with it and hope to give it away. With attractive power comes extra attention from the group, and this can feel heavy for some members. They may fantasise about escaping the spotlight. This might have to do with freedom or privacy, but it may also connect to a longing for safety and containment. Masochistic sexual fantasies from very powerful members may be one expression of this, and perhaps Gilgamesh's dream of being mastered by the hairy Wild Man Enkidu is an example.

Taboo fantasies within groups have difficulty finding expression, by definition, and we should know by now that repression leads to problematic expression. Repressed material does not stay down very well, as Cronus demonstrates. This is similar to the laws of physics with a gas: the more pressure exerted on a gas, the more violently it seeks escape from the container. So, when groups decline to talk about the attraction in the room between members, where does this energy go?

Almost certainly, one outlet is the informal power structure, in the form of extra effort to gain access to attractive members. This can and does manifest in literal underground sexual pairings in organisations (and group relations conferences). Sexuality or attractiveness may be explicitly weaponised at times, as discussed by William White (1997). He highlights a case study in which a sexual relationship emerged between an employee and his supervisor's wife during a time of conflict in both the supervisor–employee and supervisor–spouse relationships. White postulated that the sexual relationship was an act of aggression toward the supervisor rather than an act of affection for both parties involved. Here we see sexual gratification as secondary to the act of relational violence—sexuality wielded as an expression of underground power.

In a less intense form, we may see attraction used to create a favour economy, where attractive members hold extra sway over decisional matters, although it is not explicitly acknowledged. When the formal authority gives a directive, the group may first gauge the reaction of the attractive members before forming a response. Attractive members may subtly recruit others to fight battles for them. It is implied that members who cooperate will gain more approval from the attractive members.

Attractive members may tend to hold the gaze of colleagues for disproportionately long periods of time. In the Narcissus myth, when he falls in love with himself, he cannot help but stare at the pool's reflection. The eyes often follow the attractive power (although the reverse may be true in groups engaged in flight).

We intuitively feel that the eyes have power, whether it is in work meetings or a gathering of friends: we become anxious if we feel we are drawing an inappropriate amount of gaze-time, whether too little or too much. Our vision gives us important information about our environment, so where we choose to direct our gaze says much about how we value different people and objects in our environment. Leaders, therapists, and group facilitators who understand this will pick up on clues that others will miss. When someone looks at you, they are selecting you as the informational input over everything else in their environment.

Attractive members might hold others' gaze for multiple reasons. First, it becomes important for us as members to know what elicits approval from the attractive members of the group, because we do not want to act in ways that limit our access to the attractive members. We unconsciously search for clues in their body language, tone of voice, and the words they use. If we get cues from attractive members implying opposition to a certain idea, this might influence how we present our own position. This sounds manipulative on our part, and it is, although typically not on a conscious level.

If this revelation makes us uncomfortable, it might be helpful to remember that these effects are attenuated only by increasing our awareness, not by denial. If we do not want to act in this way, acknowledging the impact of lust is the first step towards gaining other behavioural paths.

A second reason that attractive members may hold our gaze is that we have to constantly reassess their attractiveness. Desirability is dynamic, not static, as mentioned above. It is partly determined by whether a trait is productive for the salient goals of the group or not, and the qualities that the group deems attractive may change over time. Additionally, we sometimes miscalculate, initially assessing a member as attractive and then later changing our opinion as we gather more information (or vice versa). Our survival and status in the group depends on our ability to reassess this information accurately in real time. When we err, it can mean that we are misreading the power landscape and wasting energy investing in unhelpful alliances.

Leaders who pay attention to which group members command disproportionate attention (or avoidance) can allow this information to inform their strategy for leading. Sometimes this might mean recruiting the powerful members to support an idea before presenting it to the group, which can increase buy-in. Other times, leaders may need to actively address or disarm unhelpful dynamics directly.

Attraction and power in a group relations conference

Aodhán Moran

The story of the Greek goddess Circe in Homer's *Odyssey* is helpful for exploring attraction and power. Like the Sirens or Cleopatra, Circe is an incarnation of the Temptress archetype, which is the shadowy opposite of the Princess. The Temptress is associated with lascivity, temptation, and unrestrained sexuality. The Temptress attracts the Hero, but ultimately complicates their quest.

> Odysseus and his men land on the island of Aeaea, home of the goddess and sorceress Circe, whose home is encircled by strangely docile lions. She invites Odysseus' men to a meal of honey, cheese, and wine which she has laced with a magical potion. On eating the meal, Odysseus' men turn into pigs.

The Temptress archetype emerged in an intergroup event at a group relations conference I attended. The conference task was to explore relations between groups of other members in real time, with a focus on problems arising from exercising authority on behalf of others. At one point, the entire membership met in one room to democratically create subgroups. Members had the option to form a subgroup, or to join a subgroup that another member was forming. I found myself torn between forming a group or joining another. Recall the push and pull of the leadership role—it is both attractive and repulsive.

From the beginning of the conference, a member, who we will refer to as Z, had been openly expressing her sexuality. She spoke in a slow, sultry rhythm. She was among the first to introduce her own sexual desires to the large group. She complimented my pectoral muscles while staring at my chest. In the intergroup event (described above) Z led the formation of a group. Upon seeing this, I disregarded any ideas of leading and joined her group.

Reflecting on my choices, I concluded that the allure of Z's free expression of sexuality played a large part in my joining. It might be said that I suffered the same fate as Odysseus' men who drank Circe's potion. Like a pig following their base instincts, I unwittingly walked a trail set by my desire without questioning my actions. While it is inevitable that unconscious forces have an influence over group formation, I found myself filled with shame and disgust.

Over the next two days, the group continued to mobilise Z to take up a leadership role. Two male members took up helper roles, tending to Z's suggestions. I was on the outside, unsure of how to engage, and I felt my body growing tired and heavy. I felt unable to speak, and my silence began to fill the room. Filled with emotion that I failed to put words to, I abruptly left the session.

Returning to the group the following day, despite my best intentions, I found myself in the same situation. There was something happening within the group that I could not contain. Put another way, the group was trying to express something indigestible through me. Rather than think productively with the group, I continued to sit in silence, effectively aborting the group's attempts at productive thinking— a destructive act.

For those unfamiliar with group relations conferences, it's important to note that I consciously had *no idea* what was happening. It felt as if I was wading through molasses. Entering into dialogue with other members seemed truly impossible. This is often the case when possessed by an affect that has not been properly integrated. It is easy to dismiss silence as nothing, but silence can be a weapon, passive-aggressively funnelling a group toward a desired end.

Applying the group-as-a-whole lens, we might ask what the group was mobilising in me. What was occurring in both our group and the wider conference that generated my response? Competition? Rebellion against the formalised female leadership? Misogyny? All of the above?

Eventually, I asked the group to help me put words to what was going on. Z asserted that I was jealous of the dynamic between her and another male group member. Much to my own amazement, this resonated deeply. I immediately felt physically lighter and more energised. The energy of the room changed. The group started to think together productively again.

In this case, unrequited desire resulted in jealousy, envy, and competition. This led me to attempt a coup of Z's leadership through sullen silence, rather than productively working with the group.

Returning to our myth:

> When Odysseus goes to rescue his men, the messenger god Hermes tells Odysseus to eat moly herb to protect himself from Circe's allure and then lunge at her when she tries to strike him with her sword. Odysseus follows Hermes' instructions and Circe immediately changes to friendly and helpful, eventually becoming Odysseus' lover, and he and his men live with her in luxury for a year.

According to Edward Edinger (1994), the moly herb was used in late antiquity to symbolise the development of consciousness. A white flower with black roots, moly was thought of as whiteness that grows out of darkness. Moly was used by the Stoics, Neoplatonists, and early Church Fathers to illustrate various ideas. On the basis of its widespread use in ancient literature, Edinger speculates that moly acted to bring the unconscious content into the realm of the conscious.

Through the moly root, Hermes grants Odysseus a means of protection against Circe's sorcery. Odysseus' newfound awareness of the Temptress' powers enables him to work with these forces, rather than being overwhelmed by them.

Like Odysseus taking the moly root from Hermes to overcome Circe's spell, conscious acknowledgement of my attraction brought the group back on task.

As we can see in both mythological and real-world examples, attraction can cause issues within group settings because it can evoke potentially divisive emotions such as jealousy, envy, rejection, competition, shame, and even ecstasy. Group relations conferences are particularly ideal training grounds for building awareness of these dynamics because there is less on the line than 'real-world' organisations. Experiencing and analysing these dynamics in a conference environment helps leaders navigate these scenarios based not just on a dry theory but through embodied experience.

* * *

We acknowledged that groups tend to avoid honest discussion about attraction in the room, and that this may often be a wise move given shorter-term group goals. This generally happens at the level of the unconscious. Finding oneself in Aphrodite's realm often leads to trouble, as seen in the tragic myths of Adonis and Hippolytus:

> The mortal Adonis charms Aphrodite only to be gored by a boar sent by Ares, one of Aphrodite's jealous lovers. In another myth, Aphrodite casts a spell on the mortal Phaedra, causing her to fall in love with her stepson, the chaste warrior Hippolytus. After Hippolytus rejects Phaedra's advances, jealousy drove her to tell her husband Theseus that Hippolytus had sexually molested her. Theseus invoked Poseidon to punish Hippolytus, after which Hippolytus was dragged to death by his own horses.

Yet in the long run, such compulsive avoidance and repression of shadow material can be quite limiting for groups and member relations. There is a deep freedom often experienced by groups that explore the topic of attraction with each other, when done properly. We touch something deep and genuine when this part of our human experience can be openly spoken. The topic is a high-risk, high-reward proposition, because the threat of relational damage upon revealing ourselves is real. If we refer back to our Norse creation myth, this is one of the ways the humans arrive. When a group contains an emotionally safe culture, and deeper member connections will help towards group goals, it may be an appropriate time for group members to explore the topic. However, we recall that dwarf work must have taken place beforehand—healthy boundaries must be in place for this topic to be navigated effectively.

We probably all have a sense of the threat of discussing attraction candidly. Naming attraction that is not reciprocated hurts, and when such a wound is dealt, one way we can protect our self-image is to project something bad on the member who spurned us, which comes with its own set of negative relational consequences. This situation is rather common, and the fear of it is likely one of the driving forces that keeps group defences up. Alternatively, if strong attraction is shared between members, but appropriate boundaries are not in place, the strong pairing that occurs may sabotage the goals of the group as well. It is typically perceived as a lower-risk option to simply avoid the topic. And this is preferred in the majority of working environments.

It is also worth acknowledging that there are multiple ecosystems for attraction within a group, and there is an economic element to attraction, as exhibited in the competition between goddesses to catalyse the Trojan War. In a group with three gay male members, there may arise competition that would not be present if there were two members, and this would be different from one gay member, etc. This phenomenon may explain why group members who share important similarities may bring up anxiety for each other. Competition for niches within the group becomes a salient problem. In the chapter on incest, we discussed suspicion of differences between members, but due to the competitive economics of attraction, there can also be elevated anxiety when members share salient strengths.

I once worked on a team with two members who both prided themselves on bringing spirituality into the work. Separately, they were often admired and seen as attractive for this quality. Yet by the end of this project there was clear discord, as neither one of them was able to fully hold the role of the spiritual one. In the Trojan War arc, when Patroclus dons Achilles' armour to lead the Myrmidons, he is killed in battle. There is only room for one Achilles. Competition deserves its own chapter, but there is clearly a link between competition and attraction.

* * *

What about self-directed lust, both on the individual and group level? It is common that instead of manifesting attraction towards the other, groups direct their attraction inward, and become egoically inflated. The Greek parable of Narcissus gives us rich material:

> Narcissus is a youth of unrivalled beauty, who attracts the love of everyone who sees him, but rejects all advances. In a glade one day, the nymph Echo, who can only recite back the words spoken by others, falls in love with him and attempts to seduce him using his own words. He rejects her, and she eventually wastes away, leaving only her voice. Nemesis, the goddess of retribution, is angered by Narcissus' rejection of Echo and lures him to a pond, where he sees and falls in love with his own reflection. Since he cannot have the object of his desire, he eventually wastes away and dies as well.

Narcissus may be the most famous example of lust in mythology, and we also see the term 'narcissism' used commonly (and liberally) to describe certain personality pathology.

From our group-as-a-whole lens in modern society, we might observe that self-lust has formed an entwined relationship with technology. Specifically, social media has become a channel and amplifier for our narcissistic tendencies. Social media serves us up a distorted reflection of ourselves. Just like Narcissus, modern humans sit and gawk at reflective screens to the point of self-harm.

Is it a coincidence that we describe social media platforms as 'Echo chambers', or is it a subconscious homage to the nymph in the Narcissus myth? Like Narcissus, we stare into our own metaphorical reflection. Our postures and physiques reflect the damage we endure. Aside from the outward effects, psychologists are only beginning to measure the negative impact that social media consumption has on our psyches, especially adolescents. The psychologist Jonathan Haidt speaks to these effects in his recorded talks. Nothing good happens when a still-undeveloped self is over-exposed to a toxic Echo chamber.

Concurrently, our society has become increasingly critical of selective narcissistic elements. It has become popular to fling the narcissist label at celebrities and social media influencers. A Google Ngram Viewer search of the term 'narcissism' demonstrates our increased usage of the term over time as a percentage of words in searchable texts (Figure 2).

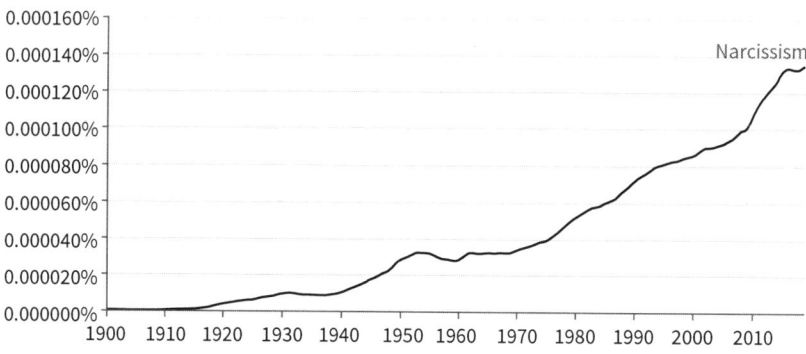

Figure 2. Graph of increased usage of the term 'narcissism'.

A golden rule, when dealing with projections, is that the things we most condemn in others are likely unintegrated within our own psyche. In this case, we might hypothesise that our internal Narcissus remains unintegrated, doing great damage, while we project him outwards.

We can also recall that Persephone was abducted as she wandered away from her entourage to pick the Narcissus flower. Something of our rejuvenative powers are pulled down into the underworld—or repressed—when we are seduced into narcissism. It is possible that we see this on a societal level, and that the activation of widespread narcissism correlates with a decline in the nourishing energies. Seduction into the Narcissus energy is a precursor to feminine archetypal energy being repressed. If we are fixated on our own reflection, we cannot show up for others. Groups that are over-inflated or self-aggrandising can alienate outsiders and may become toxic closed systems.

It is helpful for us as leaders, coaches, and facilitators to understand that the Narcissus energy presents from a wounded place. This self-focused attraction leads to death for Narcissus in the story. There is an emptiness wanting to be filled—a Lacanian lack. This type of energy is very difficult to work with in groups. We may have an instinct to confront or attempt to otherwise deflate the group, but the defence mechanisms in place for a narcissistic group often make this difficult, and it can be hard to find a way in. It feels like a cousin of addiction, and until there is a strong reckoning, the inflated or narcissistic organisation is likely to maintain its trajectory. For American car companies in the 1980s and 1990s, it took losing significant market share to Japanese manufacturers to break the spell.

CHAPTER 10

War and competition

War and conflict decorate mythical landscapes and can be said to convey something about the competition between different psychic elements within a group. As we have discussed, the Trojan War begins with the competition between goddesses discussed previously. Athena, Aphrodite, and Hera seek to win over the mortal Paris for the title of fairest.

> Prince Paris, for choosing Aphrodite as the fairest goddess, is promised Helen as a bride. He sails to Sparta, seduces her during her husband's absence, and takes her back to Troy. Menelaus, Helen's husband and the brother of King Agamemnon, is angered and recruits Greece's warlords to join him against Troy in a war that will last ten years.

The myth begins with competition between goddesses and culminates in a decade-long war that splits even the gods among themselves.

Competition always involves scarcity of a needed resource, whether actual or perceived. Paris can only crown one goddess as the fairest. That is not to say that groups cannot take a collaborative stance or work together to expand the available resources—nor does it imply competition always involves bloodshed. However, it is unavoidable that *some* resources will be limited (or perceived as limited), and some level of competition arises when the needs of multiple parties require the same limited resources. French scholar René Girard put forward that rivalry and competition stems from two peers' desire for the same object (Cayley, 2019).

In a family system, we may see an infant become jealous of his new-born sister when she gets more parental attention (a limited and valuable resource). The older child begins to act out and vie for parental attention by crying and stomping around, and if unresolved, there can be enmity between the siblings thereafter. The resources must be shared, multiplied, and/or divided up appropriately for a peaceful resolution to occur.

The alternative is a win–lose conflict. In this case, the older sibling may internalise a diminished sense of self-esteem, reorienting their expectations of getting needs met in an unhealthy way.

As any new group forms, members engage in competition for status within the group. The context, once again, determines which attributes are valued when establishing the hierarchy. On a sports team, the pecking order may be determined by athletic performance and members' understanding of the game. In a boardroom, indicators of an individual's business acumen (such as school attended, degree earned, prior business success) may play a bigger role. Many times, subconscious group drives will dominate as the determining factors of which attributes are most valued. This helps explain why some social groups seem to value traits that are not easily explainable as bringing value to the stated group goals. In group conferences, we have seen members paradoxically gain power by claiming the most disempowerment from society. This idea hearkens back to our earlier discussion of inverted hierarchies.

There are fantasies of non-competitive groups in certain political systems of thought, but anecdotally and from an organisational psychological perspective, eliminating competition is neither possible nor desirable. A lack of competition seems to undermine healthy development for both the group and individuals.

Patrick Lencioni (2002) cites an avoidance of conflict as one of the core dysfunctions in many teams, and points out that some parts of our individual psyches demand conflict in order to stay engaged. He observes that work meetings often feel meaningless because of a lack of healthy conflict. Conflict can spur positive growth and adaptation, both of which are needed survival traits for groups in a world that does not stand still. Nathaniel Branden argues that as organisational demands rise in our increasingly complex world, the most important skill for organisations to foster is adaptability—a skill that requires practice in the face of challenge and conflict. Of course, unhealthy handling of competition can do damage as well. Western culture seems to be more in touch with this side of competition's shadow.

Additionally, it is worth recognising that resources exist on a spectrum of tangibility. Examples of tangible resources include formal titles, material wealth, measurable market share, and access to preferred sexual partners. Less tangible resources may include free time, social connection, and social standing. Given this, it can sometimes be hard to discern which resources are triggering competition within or between groups. As a general rule, if we are unable to trace a group conflict to a scarce resource, it implies that we do not understand that particular conflict.

Acknowledging the competition or conflict that exists in the room tends to be experienced as taboo, possibly because bringing it to light inhibits the group fantasy from being acted out. If the group is locked into a fight reaction or a toxic pairing in service to an unconscious drive, the unconscious is likely to be frustrated by the cool, rational acknowledgement and discussion of these dynamics. It becomes hard to fight with other group members if the conflict is also being actively discussed, and this is usually a good thing for the group's movement towards its conscious goals. As Lencioni points out, naming and resolving conflict quickly and efficiently is a defining characteristic of high-functioning teams. Facilitators should anticipate some form of resistance from the unconscious as they bring the dynamics into the light.

When we imagine conflict, we may fantasise that it originates at the tops of organisations, or at least takes place in a clean, linear fashion between two entities. We watch television dramas about business moguls enacting planned hostile takeovers, or mediaeval royalty executing nuanced schemes to conquer enemies. In the popular series *Game of Thrones*, the most powerful characters act as movers of chess pieces, often anticipating events far in advance. The conflicts are portrayed as the result of individual conscious motives.

In reality, conflict is typically messy and involves unconscious group motivations. Leaders are probably more likely to be swept along for the ride than to have planned for the conflicts that grip the group. The Trojan War does not stem from well-laid plans of queens or kings; rather, Discord tosses the golden apple labelled 'for the fairest' into the midst of the Olympians. A prince and a king's brother find themselves in competition for Helen after an impulsive promise is made by a goddess. All other major players, including the great heroes such as Achilles and Odysseus (and even the gods), are pulled into the conflict as if it were a rip tide. The group mobilises the major players without their planning, or even their consent. The group exerts a strong magnetism on all members. Members are used by the group psyche, many times in ways that they might resent at some level.

Another tempting fantasy about group conflict is that it is neatly contained within an episode or two. In reality, conflicts may bubble over into outright hostility, but often, we see a dragging out of tensions, where passive guerrilla warfare drags group relationships and productivity into a quagmire. The group psyche that manifests a conflict does so for a reason, even if it is unconscious. Groups are skilled at defending useful conflicts from premature resolution. Likewise, the roles that members take up in the face of conflict have staying power as long as they are providing value towards the goals of the group unconscious.

The Trojan War lasted for ten years, stemming from one offence. This is typical for groups, but also avoidable under most circumstances when competent leaders take corrective action. Wise leaders might start with the question, 'How is this conflict serving the group?'

From a reader's perspective, the Trojan War has heroes on both sides. It is not a simple us-vs-them narrative, in which one party holds the badness, and we are able to clearly identify with the Greeks or Trojans. The gods are split, and we see admirable traits and disturbing ones on both sides of the line. It is not courage on the part of the victors that finally wins the day, but trickery and subterfuge. The victors sack and burn Troy, and the majority of the heroes die during the course of the war (or will die before they return home). This gives us a flavour of the blurred lines and messiness involved with group conflict.

And yet, we can also trace the destruction of Troy to the creation of Rome, through Aeneas' journey thereafter. In this sense, we should conceptualise conflict as a potent group force that can be destructive, yet also may underpin new beginnings and potentialities for groups.

CHAPTER 11

Scapegoating

We opened the book with a scapegoating example from a group of boys in wilderness therapy. Scapegoating tends to be one of the clearest illustrations of group dynamics. Although the example chosen involved a group with younger members, this pattern is not limited to therapeutic adolescent groups. High-level teams of professionals are also prone to invoking a scapegoat dynamic. We discussed the idea of metaphorical murder in a previous chapter, and certainly there can be significant overlap between murder and scapegoating. We treat scapegoating as a related but more narrow concept.

The term scapegoat reaches far back into history. The scapegoat concept appeared in the Book of Leviticus: a goat was ritually 'filled' with the sins of the village and banished to the wilderness, cleansing the wrongdoings of the people. Scapegoating rituals emerged in Ancient Greece, where a community would select an ugly member, stone them, and then take them to the borders of the city in hopes that they would carry the sins of the community away. It has become the common term for any situation in which a group projects undesirable qualities onto one member, subgroup, or external entity in order to consolidate blame and avoid accountability.

Strangely, the Ancient Greek word pharmakós, which translates to *scapegoat*, is closely related to phármakon, which translates to *medicine* (Crimi, 2021). The etymology of the term points to an intuitive grasp of the medicinal power of the scapegoat dynamic. William White (1997) observed that both internal and external scapegoating serves the system by temporarily diffusing internal conflict. René Girard believed humans form community through channelling violence towards sacrificial victims (Cayley, 2019). We see this in the trope of the foundational murder repeated throughout myth: Romulus and Remus, Cain and Abel. Similarly, a shared orientation against an outside entity can have a net positive short-term effect on member relations. Damon Albarn of the band Gorillaz wrote: 'This storm brings strange loyalties'. We are reminded of Frans de Waal's observations of chimps in the Arnhem zoo: When intra-group tensions reached a certain point, they would let off steam by screaming at the neighbouring lions and cheetahs (De Waal, 2005).

We see this in the lead up to the Trojan War. Odysseus advises Agamemnon to require all of Helen's suitors to agree to defend Helen's honour in the future in order to be eligible for her hand. Menelaus and many of the other Greek heroes are in conflict for the hand of Helen prior to the war, yet unite together against Troy when she is abducted by Paris. This cements otherwise acrimonious relationships within the Greek ranks. Peace based on an external enemy is not usually in the long-term best interest of a group—these groups are prone to self-destruction down the line. The smaller internal conflicts may be set aside temporarily, but if they are not resolved, they will surface at inconvenient times when a crisis of sufficient magnitude is not present. It behoves leaders to identify Odysseus' pact when it arises.

Through our work with groups, we have seen two distinct categories of scapegoats within groups. The first category is the scapegoat onto which the group projects psychic material and then kills off, metaphorically or literally. This first type fits in with the historical origin of the phrase more neatly. The goat is sacrificed or pushed out into the wilderness.

The second category of scapegoat is made to hold group projection as well, but the group becomes immensely invested in keeping this member around as a perpetual receptacle for unwanted psychic material. They stick around.

The Greek myth of Atlas serves as a metaphor for this second type of scapegoating dynamic in groups:

> After supporting the failed Titan rebellion against Olympus, the Titan Atlas is punished by Zeus, who forces Atlas to hold the sky upon his shoulders for eternity. It is said that anyone who purposefully accepts the burden will bear it forever, or until they can trick another into accepting it. He remains stuck at the western edge of the world, bearing his burden, until Hercules eventually approaches him for help in gaining the golden apples that Atlas' daughters tend.
>
> Atlas is able to convince Hercules to hold the sky temporarily while he fetches the apples, and then attempts to trick Hercules into accepting the burden for eternity by offering to deliver the golden apples for him. Hercules pretends to agree, on the condition that Atlas takes the burden back for a moment so that he can adjust his cloak for padding. Upon handing the sky back to Atlas, Hercules takes the apples and escapes.

Atlas' fate gives us a feel for the scapegoat, because his role is both a burden but also strangely valuable for the group. Atlas holds up the sky, and in our everyday groups the scapegoat offers value to the group in a profound way that is rarely recognised.

The myth tells us something of the difficulty of escaping a scapegoat dynamic as well. In the story, Atlas is able to hand over the burden (or role) to Hercules for a brief moment, yet Hercules tricks him into taking on the burden again. In group relations work, we often see the group audition members for certain roles that end up not sticking. The role didn't stick to Hercules, and Atlas lands back in it. This gives us a sense of what is meant by Bion's idea of *role valence* (Vazard, 2022).

We may find ourselves taking on similar roles in different groups throughout our lives, and this is likely because of our valence, or proclivity to fit a certain archetypal role for the group. Our valence may change as we evolve and increase awareness about our own personal patterns. There is a connection here to what Lacan (2016) calls our individual 'symptom', *the way in which we find our enjoyment in the unconscious.*

In my early work with group relations and in organisational life, I found myself taking on the persecutor role and spearheading conflict within groups. As time went on, I was able to recognise these tendencies in myself and avoid being used by the group in this way (to an extent—the symptom remains). Of course, as I stepped out of this role, others seemed to step in and fill the void, and the total amount of group conflict never seemed to decrease somehow. Although I no longer held Ares, the god of war, he was still present with the crowd. Groups tend to fill archetypal vacuums in order to meet the desires of the unconscious.

As we see in the Atlas myth, there is sometimes an element of trickery involved with attempts to escape a role. Moving the group scapegoat projection away from oneself requires some sleight of hand, and is easiest when another target presents itself. This is not a pretty thing to say, but experience tells us that it is true. As we discussed in previous chapters, it is possible for groups to reclaim the shadow material that they have given to the scapegoat, but there are reasons that groups will usually resist this process, especially when a ready vessel exists for scapegoating.

One of the most vicious and obvious scapegoating dynamics I have ever seen took place at a Boston residential groups conference. Over the course of five days, I watched an intelligent and sensitive therapist slowly degrade into a clumsy, belligerent clown of a man. He was White, middle-aged, gay, and seemed politically liberal. On the first day, he made an ambiguous comment about politics that could have been interpreted as derogatory towards Barack Obama, and several White women expressed offence. He took a defensive stance, giving them something more to push against, and the group-as-a-whole began the process of eating him alive. I remember thinking, 'Well, I'm glad it isn't going to be me'.

As the anger towards him escalated and crystallised, he began to stammer and interrupt more often. He became decreasingly aware of his body and others' personal space. He would accidentally drape his hand too close to a woman's groin sitting behind him, or carelessly stand within inches of others while talking loudly. These oversights infuriated group members all the more. By the end of the conference, some members would begin to cry and shake within seconds of him speaking. These were otherwise intelligent professionals, mind you, at a Boston College retreat centre.

At one point, he made an angry exit after a series of heated public arguments with other members. When he left the room, the group was suddenly lost. An awkwardness hung in the air. Whatever grace we expected to come with his departure did not materialise. If anything, it seemed that members felt greater anxiety. The group was saved when he sheepishly re-entered the room minutes later, as if he had been summoned back by the group-as-a-whole. On some level, it seemed that the group needed him to hold that scapegoat role. It did something for all of us.

One fascinating aspect of the scapegoat dynamic is the readiness with which certain group members seem to nominate themselves to fill the role. On the surface, the role of the scapegoat sounds miserable—scapegoats are often ridiculed, demeaned, and blamed for anything and everything that goes wrong. Yet if we can admit that leadership roles are sometimes seen in a distortedly positive light, we can say the opposite is true of the scapegoat role. There is some hidden value in the role, implied by the readiness with which certain members cooperate with the role and the tenacity with which they seem to cling to it.

For one thing, members who hold the scapegoat role often gain extra attention from the group. The scapegoat may be disliked on a level, but they *matter*. A scapegoat is seen by the group, albeit through a darkened lens.

Also, the scapegoat may feel an easing of the responsibility to perform, since the group typically projects an incompetence onto the holder of the scapegoat archetype. They will often not be burdened with a high amount of responsibility in the traditional sense. Yet we should note that sometimes groups prepare for a scapegoat dynamic by overloading a specific member with responsibility, such that they are likely to fail. Alternatively, a group may load the scapegoat mantle onto a member who fills an essential function in the group, perhaps in an attempt to reduce the person's self-worth and exert some control, belying the fear that this member might abandon the group. In essence, impressing upon the important member, 'You can't leave, no one else would have you'.

Scapegoating is slightly more nuanced than member assassination, which carries with it a repressive intent. Because of the value they contribute at a psychic level, the group often protects its scapegoat at times, especially from external threats. We may hear an older sibling say 'Nobody messes with my little brother except me', and groups often seem to feel similarly about their scapegoats.

A key observation in support of the archetypal nature of group dynamics is the staying power of a scapegoat pattern. The role is bigger than the individual member who holds it. If a group has engaged in scapegoating, it does not generally matter whether the individual member leaves the group; the dynamic persists with a new target. The group will recruit another member to step in and take the vacant role. Someone needs to 'hold the sky'. This hand-off can happen surprisingly quickly when a prior scapegoat leaves the system, as our opening story from the wilderness illustrates.

Astute group members may recognise that there is a critical period after such a member leaves in which it is wise to lie low, from an individual's perspective. Members feel it and may acknowledge it in the hallways between meetings: 'Who's next?' In these moments, auditions are taking place for the next scapegoat. The group has been meeting its need to project its undesirable characteristics—incompetence, weakness, ugliness—on a particular member, but it can and will move those projections onto a new member when necessary, if the material is not integrated.

Leaders and group facilitators may be able to take advantage of this window after a scapegoat leaves to address the dynamic with the group and move towards psychic integration. There may be two reasons why this window presents such an opportunity:

First, in the presence of an intact scapegoat, the group has reached a kind of equilibrium. Any attempt to confront the actual group pattern will likely be met with resistance, because it will require a large amount of emotional and psychic energy, as opposed to continuing with the benefits and momentum of utilising the scapegoat. Doing the integrating work is not much of a bargain in the eyes of the group unconscious. The group would be giving up something delicious. Intervention is not impossible, but it is difficult.

Yet when a scapegoat leaves, the system is thrown temporarily out of equilibrium. Reintegration of the projected shadow material offers an option for returning to stability, albeit of a different kind. Moving the scapegoating projection onto a new candidate takes energy as well, so, by comparison to the previous equilibrium, it may be less 'work' to begin integrating.

Second, when a scapegoat departs, and before any other member starts to take up the role, the group may be willing to acknowledge that no member *currently* appears worthy of holding all the blame for the group. The implication of stating this explicitly is that when the group does start to recruit a new scapegoat, it can more plausibly be explained as a group pattern rather than an individual shortcoming. The unhealthy pattern is laid bare for all to see more clearly. A facilitator or manager might comment, 'It's interesting that we were in agreement that everyone here has something to contribute, but now we are seeing some blaming behaviour from the group again. Did something change in the individuals, or is this more likely a pattern for us?'

We might also become curious about what member traits correlate with the taking up of a scapegoat role. In our experience, a scapegoat always carries anxiety, or they will not have a valence for the role. Anxiety acts as a kind of glue between the role and the individual. Members with a calm, relaxed demeanour do not have the 'stickiness' required. The group may audition them for the role in some unconscious sense (as Hercules held the sky for a short time), but they will likely fail to satisfy the group. Anxiety is what inspires a defensive stance in a scapegoat candidate, which allows the group something to further push against. Displays of anxiety belie an insecure sense of self, which suggests a more ready canvas on which group projections may take hold. This manifests in different ways, such as the chosen member 'not feeling heard', or being 'misunderstood'. For leaders and group facilitators, it is important to pay close attention to this type of language from members, as it almost certainly implies the presence of a relevant group dynamic.

Lastly, we should note that the scapegoat role varies in appearance. It is not monochromatic. There are various shades and hues of this phenomenon, depending on the social context—specifically, which energies the group is mobilised to disown. Just as we previously noted that a leader is tolerated to the extent that they serve the group unconscious drive, a scapegoat is similarly activated based on the dominant urge of the group.

For example, an aggressive, stoic person may fit a saviour role on the lacrosse field, and then fit a scapegoat role in a therapy group later the same day. Different archetypes are celebrated (or disowned) based on different group goals. The valence of the member for certain archetypes contributes to the likelihood that they will be recruited into that role, but there is a dance between context, valence, and the valences of other members present. After all, it took Hercules, another physically strong mythic figure, to even be a candidate to take away Atlas' burden.

CHAPTER 12

The great floods and groupthink

We have touched on water symbolism, but great flood stories deserve a deeper dive. Epic floods appear in many different myths across time and cultures and tend to share some commonalities.

The 'warning' is one such commonality. Noah, given a premonition by God, survives the great Biblical flood by building a ship and bringing pairs of each animal aboard. Utnapishtim, warned by the wisdom goddess Ea, survives the Babylonian flood in a ship as well. Prometheus advises Deucalion to prepare a chest to float in with his wife to survive Zeus' flood. In the Indian lore, Manu is warned by a great fish of the coming disaster. In the Aztec version, Tlaloc warns the devout couple Tata and Nena. Two Incan brothers are warned by their llamas of the incoming flood (Bierlein, 1995).

The obvious common theme in flood stories is the rising water from a divine source. Jung believed that water in mythology stands for the unconscious, the unknown, or the depths of the soul (Jung, 1991). Water is life-giving and also potentially deadly. In the context of group mythopoetic study, the coming of the floodwaters can be seen as an emergence of shadow material in the group psyche. The word flood implies that it is not a measured exploration of darkness, it is a danger-ous clearing-out event and an existential threat. From the group lens, the flood could be a fitting symbol for the phenomena of groupthink or mob mania.

Yale psychologist Irving Janis originally described the concept of groupthink in 1971. Groupthink occurs when tight-knit group members become over-identified with the group. A strong, insulated belief sys-tem develops without room for dissent. This leads to radicalisation and sometimes horrific group actions. Group members become enthralled with the importance of the group vision (and often a charismatic leader) and adopt delusions of group infallibility. Intense scapegoating of an outside entity is often involved. Groupthink involves a dimming of the consciousness on a group level and is much more common than we are comfortable acknowledging. We can again reference our Shinto sun goddess myth. By disallowing any dissenting viewpoints to be peace-fully discussed, groups effectively push Amaterasu into her cave while the malicious ocean god Susanoo is permitted to cause havoc. If we return to the lens of the Norse creation myth, groupthink amounts to a great southern blaze, in which group members' individuality is con-sumed by the group's larger identity, and the fire blazes out of control. The Salem witch-trials are a real-life example. The Holocaust is another. Certain strains of nationalism can be this. But we also see it in corpora-tions and start-ups.

We can currently identify signs of groupthink in both political parties in the US. The characters in the myths get warnings from Prometheus, Ea, or a great fish. We are getting such warnings from some academics and social scientists. Comedians, holding the sacred irreverent Jester archetype, are also drawing our attention to certain social issues.

Interestingly, the flood stories typically have a designated survivor (or two). With a group-as-a-whole lens applied, we imagine these char-acters as a piece of preserved consciousness within a group under the thrall. This may manifest as an individual expressing scepticism at great cost to his/her social standing. During the flood, this energy may be sealed up in a ship and repressed, yet it is also the force behind the renewal after the waters recede.

The idea of *finding land* after the waters have receded is an important theme in these stories. If the waters represent an uprising of unintegrated psychic group material, then finding land is a return to the integrated and solid. In his book *Parallel Myths*, J. F. Bierlein (1995) points out that in the Algonquin, Cree, Mesopotamian, and Christian flood myths, a raven is sent out to find land—a black bird that feasts on carrion. It is as though integrating the Jungian shadow plays an important role in our return to sanity. Perhaps Nelson Mandela was thinking along similar lines when he assumed power at the end of the Apartheid era in South Africa, when he allowed for amnesty of perpetrators under the old system, if they testified and disclosed their actions. Taking an honest look at the damage done is raven-work.

Another element common to flood myths—and an under-represented factor in leadership and group dynamics literature—is divine disgust. If we say that attraction presents a strong taboo, then we can say the same for disgust. Groups may engage in intra-group conflict at times, but rarely will outright expressions of disgust between members rise to the surface. Disgust is not to be discussed. The conversation around it is generally not pretty. Even more than attraction and competition, feelings of disgust are typically kept underground during group relations conferences.

In these flood myths, disgust often comes from above, whether it is Zeus, Yahweh, or Enlil. Moreover, we see from the flood myth that disgust evokes a massive, world-changing action from the gods. It is a horrible set of events that follows disgust. The flood stories reside in our group consciousness and hang in the air as a threat to group members.

Group members are usually highly motivated to avoid disgust of the leader or the group-as-a-whole. Again, we can trace our instincts here back to ancestral survival. Those who elicited disgust from peers were less likely to have access to resources or find a mate. Corroborating this is the typical response we see from the recipient of disgust: they anxiously act to remedy the situation and improve their group standing.

Thus, disgust can be used in dark, manipulative ways by toxic leaders, and this is often a part of the groupthink formula. Dr Jordan Peterson (2014) has postulated that leaders such as Hitler were high in a personality trait he calls disgust sensitivity, a trait that correlates with black-and-white moral thinking (or splitting). However, expressing disgust is certainly appropriate at times. When group members act unacceptably, the expression of some disgust will attach a negative emotional experience to their actions. This shapes behaviour more quickly than a reasoned argument or guideline, and seems to set the boundaries into the nervous systems of group members more fully. When unhealthy behaviour or harmful ideation is expressed by group members, a slight curling of the lips and a raised eyebrow can create a deeper impression than any formal admonition. Leaders and facilitators should keep an eye on who in such groups is authorised to express disgust.

Further, there may be times in which a lack of expressed disgust by leadership feels disturbing to group members who, at some level, understand they (or other members) are not performing appropriately. It can imply a dearth of conviction or self-esteem on the part of a leader. It may undermine the felt importance of the group task. Teams and leaders that have a clear picture of excellence tend not to tolerate inappropriate behaviour. Conversely, leaders who permit inappropriate behaviour communicate the absence of a clear vision, or at least a lack of passion for actualising it.

This of course flies in the face of New Age leadership culture, which has trended more towards what Bly (1997) refers to as the Sibling Society: flattened hierarchies, horizontal relations with managers and leaders, and an emphasis on compassion even at the expense of accountability. In effect, there is a fantasy that the household can operate with only brothers and sisters, and that the parental role (i.e. hierarchical authority) is no longer required. This relates back to our compulsive anger towards authority that we discussed in the hierarchy chapter.

There also exists a fantasy within Newer Age therapeutic organisations that the treatment team must gently hold any and all of a client's behaviours with warmth and politeness. In an attempt to apply humanistic principles, the treatment team becomes an ineffectual cardboard cut-out, uttering meaningless niceties—even when a client is abusive or displays bullying behaviors towards others in the milieu. In these organisations, it is frowned upon to say 'ew' at any level. Instead of the client bumping against reality in a container that might allow for meaningful processing of the experience, the whole thing is ignored and therefore validated as appropriate behaviour, leaving the client underprepared for experiences in the real world. What is meant to be a 'safe container' becomes a fake container. Staff in such organisations are at higher risk of burnout since the quiet ask is that they show up wearing a false saint mask.

This is a misapplication of the principle of unconditional regard and likely damages trust at some level. In essence, the argument there is that it would be harmful for a client to experience a full authentic human relationship (and this may be true in some instances—but should not be the default stance). There is room for expression of disgust/disapproval within a therapeutic relationship, although context plays a role. Compassion for the person needs to be preserved, even when disapproval of the behaviour is warranted. It requires skill, but can be a valuable opportunity to hold up a mirror for clients.

The Drama Triangle

In some ways, the material in this chapter—Karpman's Drama Triangle (1968)—offers the most compelling and efficient framework for many group dynamic situations. One risk with the Drama Triangle lens is that the temptation may be to overuse it. It is applicable, revealing, and practical. We include it later on in the book in the hope that readers will have an understanding of some other tools as well.

Hippolyta's myth gives us an appropriate metaphor for Karpman's framework:

> For Hercules' ninth labour, he is tasked to retrieve the magical girdle from Hippolyta, the queen of the Amazons. Upon meeting Hercules, Hippolyta receives him kindly and even willingly offers the girdle. However, the goddess Hera spreads the rumour among the Amazons that Hercules is abducting their queen, so they arm themselves and attack Hercules and his crew. Hercules, concluding that Hippolyta has betrayed him, slays her and makes off with the girdle.

What started as a peaceful meeting turns into a bloody misunderstanding. The Amazons step in to rescue Hippolyta, Hercules becomes defensively violent, and the strong Hippolyta becomes a victim. In the story, Hera's misinformation catalyses the tragedy. The roles are born from a falsehood.

Family systems therapists often refer to Stephen Karpman's 'Drama Triangle', published in 1968. The model consists of three roles, and the idea is that these three roles are often invoked by members of a system to play out a certain type of drama (Figure 3).

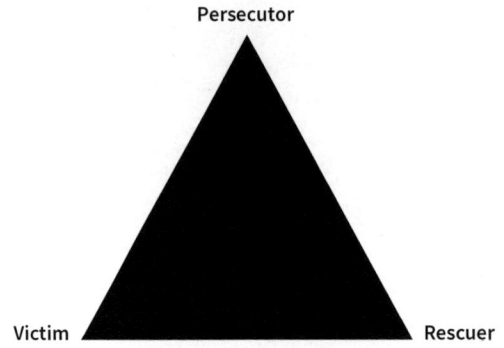

Figure 3. Stephen Karpman's Drama Triangle.

Victims subscribe to the story that they are innocent targets of injustice at the hands of the persecutor. The victim's mantra is, 'poor me'. Persecutors blame the victim, and their mantra is, 'it's all your fault'. Both the victim and the persecutor point fingers, but there is a different flavour between them. A persecutor holds the fantasy of confidence and competence, whereas a victim holds the fantasy of helpless innocence and a lack of responsibility. The line between victim and persecutor is often a thin one, however, and the roles can reverse under proper circumstances.

Rescuers come to the aid of the victim. They say, 'Let me fix this for you', or 'I will protect you from the bad man/woman'. While this behaviour may seem virtuous on the surface, in the context of the Drama Triangle it enables the victim's weakness and reinforces the villain narrative of the persecutor. Stepping into a rescuer role is an unhealthy way that some group members assuage their own feelings of anxiety, shame, or worthlessness.

Each role depends on the existence of the others, which implies that a leader or therapist might disarm the dynamic by starting with any of the three members (or subgroups) involved. Of course, other members are often eager to jump into vacated roles in the Drama Triangle. Groups, like nature, abhor a vacuum. Also, the system as a whole is likely to resist efforts to disarm the dynamic, and an intervening therapist might find themselves recruited into the Drama Triangle as a participant.

On a surface level, each of these roles seems to have some obvious drawbacks. Yet, as is a common theme in this work, we can identify seductive qualities in each as well.

Benefits of the victim role include a reduction of responsibility and an increase in sympathy from other members. There is a kind of specialness achieved in the victim role. Additionally, projecting the bully outward onto a perceived persecutor relieves the victim from owning certain unwanted qualities, such as aggression or anger. As victims, we do not have to examine our own actions or attitudes if a convincing villain can hold all the *badness*.

The persecutor benefits from disowning weakness and incompetence onto the victim. There is a kind of power in playing the villain. As villains, we are not ignored. We must be reckoned with. We do not see ourselves as villains; rather, we are fighting for an important cause and the victim is sabotaging our efforts.

The rescuer gets to live the fantasy of themselves as a virtuous caretaker. As rescuers, we claim moral superiority without sacrificing any sense of our own empowerment. A pernicious side effect is that we become invested in keeping the victim weak, since these benefits would disappear if the victim were to embrace their own capability. It is a parasitic relationship dressed up as compassion.

This is not to say that all helping action stems from such a dynamic. Some types of helping fall into the toxic rescuer category, but not all. When helping actions are motivated by relieving anxiety or shame on the part of the rescuer, toxic rescuing is likely to occur. Alas, rescuers (or anyone stuck in a group role) will not be reliable reporters of their deeper motivations, as they are of course unconscious to them.

When their identity is wound up in the protector role, they must find ways to ensure that these groups continue to need protecting. It is not in the victim's best interest to have the dynamic perpetuated, yet the rescuer is invested in just that. In Hippolyta's story, it is the Amazons rushing to rescue her who end up creating the danger, leading to her death. A part of us dies when we accept the victim role.

We call this situation a group dynamic because it has more to do with the magnetic roles that develop than the objective reality of who did what to whom. Victimhood is a mentality that exists independently of actual injustice. We can endure abuse and not adopt a victim mentality. Or we can don the victim role when we have not actually endured injustice, or when the actual injury is miniscule. Likewise, we can engage in the rescuer role when no one actually needs saving. We can certainly be perceived as a villain when no real wrongdoing has occurred on our part. And abuse can occur without the group vilifying the bad actor. In our experience with groups, these roles only correlate loosely with actual member behaviours.

In Celtic lore, the Nemedian people pay two-thirds of their crop to their oppressive neighbours, the Fomorians. This fits somewhat with our idea of projections in a model containing three roles (victim, persecutor, and rescuer). To be a victim, you must give away the other two parts of yourself via projection. The Celtic myth also speaks to the dynamic nature of the model. Eventually, the Nemedians rise up and attack the Fomorians. As mentioned earlier, the victim steps into a persecutor role rather easily.

Race relations in the US is a sensitive topic, but we can see evidence of shifting roles in the Drama Triangle. In the past, violent criminality was emphasised as a characteristic of Black men, in the form of a damaging stereotype. In the summer of 2020, following the killing of George Floyd, society seemed to be aggressively auditioning the police for the persecutor role instead.

'Defund the Police' and 'All Cops Are Bastards' trended on social media, and we can imagine that defunding is the equivalent of castration in a capitalist society. While any example of police misconduct or abuse nationwide is currently highlighted in the news, there is very little discussion of alleviating crime within minority communities in most circles at the time of this writing, which affects far more minority families by the numbers. Using the group-as-a-whole lens, we should pay special attention to the conversations that a group is *not* willing to have, as this implies some sort of avoidance. And more importantly, something important and potentially healing to the group often lies just on the other side of taboo.

Facilitators, coaches, and therapists may key in on these types of dynamics and on some level sense the danger around naming it directly. Naming the dynamic bluntly often elicits deep self-righteous anger and resentment. You become another persecutor. The narratives are strong, and the emotional advantages of acting out the roles is powerful. Groups will push back on this in order to preserve the patterns that serve them in some way.

When a Drama Triangle is activated, for example, rescuers will eschew data that compromises the perceived innocence of the victim, because this undermines the narrative, and by extension, the value gained from the rescuer role. The fantasy of total innocence for the victim must be maintained; it is facts that must go. And it is not just innocence that must be upheld; weakness must also be given convincingly to the victim, regardless of their capabilities. In the myth, Hippolyta is a strong warrior queen who is not the type that one normally expects to need saving.

When the Drama Triangle is present, members may sense that they must decide whether they will engage as a rescuer, victim, or persecutor. The neutral middle ground is rapidly eaten away until it is no longer perceptible by the group psyche.

Hippolyta's story also gives us a sense of the order in which the events take place. Hercules exists in harmony with her until Hera gets involved. Although brash and aggressive in other myths, he is getting along fine until a narrative of villainy is promulgated. We tend to believe that our narratives reflect relationships as they are, but in reality our narratives also create the quality of relationships. In our society, the media may play the role of Hera at times, inciting fear that leads to the crystallisation of the Drama Triangle roles. This applies to news outlets on both sides of the political continuum in today's world.

The Drama Triangle is not an inevitable dynamic that develops in all groups. It is an unhealthy dynamic and can be avoided. If these roles have been cast, there is projection happening. Working effectively with a group engaged in the Drama Triangle requires diffusing the dynamic, not figuring out who is the real perpetrator or getting enough justice for the victim. This is not to say that pursuing justice is never important—but it is not the solution to resolving a group dynamic.

The existence of the Drama Triangle should be addressed because it harms members and jeopardises the longer-term goals and relationships of the group. This does not mean ignoring the actions of bad actors, nor 'turning the other cheek' indiscriminately. We can be honest about our group unconscious patterns without endorsing the overall systemic architecture or a specific bad actor's deeds.

CHAPTER 14

Sabotage in organisations

After Troy falls, Odysseus and his men begin a long journey home, filled with misadventures. After escaping the Cyclops's island, they encounter Aeolus, the keeper of the winds. They stay on his island for a month, and upon departing, Aeolus gives Odysseus a skin containing all the winds except the west wind, thus making for an easy voyage home. Riding favourable winds, Odysseus and his crew quickly navigate to within sight of his home, Ithaca. At this moment Odysseus falls asleep from exhaustion, and his men open the skin of winds, believing it to be wine or treasure. As the skin opens, it releases all of the winds, blowing them all the way back to Aeolus' island, where he refuses to help them further.

In our observations of organisations pursuing goals, it is not uncommon for the leader to fall asleep within sight of home, nor for the crew to open the proverbial wineskin before the ship touches shore. This is the team that breaks into conflict when success seems within reach. Groups find clever ways to sabotage themselves when the unconscious desires a different outcome—or when success feels threatening in some way. Success is not free. It carries with it demands of the group, and has a profound effect on the group identity in ways that can endanger certain fantasies; fantasies of disowning responsibility. Thus, the group psyche may orchestrate clever failures that keep groups falling short of their stated goals. Putting the leadership to sleep, according to our myth, is the first step in such a process.

There is also the interesting piece about returning to Aeolus' island, where Odysseus received the gift originally. The contained winds are meant as a gift, yet become a liability for the men. It speaks to the idea that our gifts may also become painful burdens. Robert Bly (1990) comments that a man's genius lies next to his wound. If we turn the phrase, then we find that our deepest wounds or liabilities may be found adjacent to our gifts. Wise leaders might ask, 'How might the group's talents be mobilised in unhealthy ways?' In group relations conferences, for example, it is common for highly educated group members to use abstraction and philosophy to avoid latent conflict present in the room. Visualising such threats beforehand makes recognition easier in the moment, when the crew is seeking to open the wineskin.

The idea that a gift may be a liability for leaders converges well with the psychological study of leadership. Often a worker is promoted because s/he has performed well in his/her current position. On the face of it, this seems like a reasonable outcome, and a defensible criterion for promotion. These types of leaders thrived in the past through their high level of competency. Yet, competency at one level of an organisation does not imply competency at the next hierarchical level. The skills required of a manager are not the same as those required of a frontline worker, for example.

Leadership is about relationships and balancing big-picture decisions, and the best leaders are not always those who were the best in lower hierarchical roles. Leaning on their previous skill sets can become a limiting crutch, and potentially an obstacle to learning a new way of operating. Many of these ilk turn into overly critical micromanagers who burn out in leadership roles. Like Odysseus, they may find that the gift of the winds on the island may become a liability at sea. Returning to the island where the gift was given cannot remedy the situation, though many leaders long for a return to previous levels of responsibility.

So we are left with this: The leader fell asleep, the winds were unleashed, and the homecoming was sabotaged. Self-sabotage is discussed in-depth in the context of individual psychology, in works such as Nathaniel Branden's *Six Pillars of Self-Esteem* (1995). If we do not believe ourselves worthy of an honour, it is often easier to undermine our success than attempt to live up to the level of responsibility it demands. The unconscious may opt to pre-emptively fail rather than wait in fear for failure to surprise us. We crash-land the plane into the ocean for fear of running out of gas above the mountains.

In groups, a similar effect can occur, and with broader implications. Group-sabotage occurs when the group-as-a-whole acts to undermine the group's stated goals, in service to an unstated or unconscious goal. We've discussed group failures resulting from arrogant avoidance and groupthink, and the lens of group-sabotage allows us a different framework that might more fully explain some situations. Again, these are not mutually exclusive concepts. Groups utilise these various unconscious reactions in ways that systematically undermine the completion of group goals.

For example, a lack of due-diligence and integrity by the US banks in 2008 hints at arrogant avoidance, and contributed to the housing crisis. Similarly, internal pressure for shortcuts and an aloofness to risk reportedly contributed to NASA's Challenger disaster (Vaughan, 2016). These are highly visible collapses, but the impact of most organisational self-sabotage goes under the radar: unrealised profit, lack of worker engagement, cultures of mediocrity, and premature departures of talented leaders.

And of course, it is not simply the leader as a single entity that explains leadership and culture failure. The group-as-a-whole has a large part to play in such situations. Warren Bennis (1976) touches on some of this material in his book *The Unconscious Conspiracy*. He asserts that loyal subordinates are often guilty of unintentionally conspiring to pull the leader into the mundane and routine. Such leaders burn out or fail, as they neglect the visionary elements needed from a leader. Members of such a system become dissatisfied, and the leaders are often where fingers get pointed.

I worked in a therapeutic organisation that had become so complex through its myriad of rules and processes that culture and retention suffered horribly. The meaning of the work was lost in a sea of procedures and minutiae. The already difficult work of direct-care therapy was made unbearable by the litany of added burdens.

Of course, each individual who had contributed to the mess had done so with good intentions. It was not the case that any single person or rule was irrational; each addition to the system had made a kind of sense when it was implemented. Yet the overall result was damaging to the organisation. A teenage client of this organisation noted, 'Every solution has its problems'. In Polynesian mythology, the demigod Maui endeavours to lift the sky to create more space for his people, but as a result, shortens the daylight hours (Westervelt, 1910). And in the Mesopotamian myth, when Gilgamesh breaks the stone golems who might have helped him in his quest, he is told by the boatman Urshanabi, 'With your own hands you have made the crossing harder' (Ferry, 1993, p. 60).

Whenever this trend is manifested by an organisation on such a consistent basis and without stated intention, we can guess that there is a subconscious drive at play. Remember, we assume that there are no coincidences in group behaviour. If a behaviour is taking place, there is a drive for what the behaviour is producing.

While there is no awareness of this type of process happening among the group members, there is extensive unconscious cooperation on their part that supports the process. In my experience with the organisation described above, not only was the complicit behaviour occurring, but the organisation was extremely resistant to change course. This is despite the programme director being open to hearing feedback about the system and earnest in wanting improvement. The unconscious organisational forces at work are powerful and deeply rooted. This can be thought of as a universal truth in our study of groups.

CHAPTER 15

The crisis compulsion

There is a subcategory of group-sabotage that deserves special attention. I call this delineation the *crisis compulsion*. Crisis compulsion occurs when a group acts unconsciously to perpetually create crises for itself to manage. One might conclude that Odysseus' sequence of misadventures hints at a crisis compulsion, for example. Again, if a group constantly encounters something, we can guess that some part of the group psyche desires the encounters.

The term *crisis*, on the surface, carries a negative connotation. We expect that crises drastically increase stress and that everyone in any organisation would agree that they should be avoided. Yet paradoxically, certain types of organisational crises can alleviate anxiety or inspire positive excitement, especially for insecure leaders. When a crisis occurs, the value hierarchy for leadership skill shifts. Abstract, long-term thinking takes a back seat to action. The demand for elbow grease increases dramatically.

In many emergency situations, the requirements of a leader become more clarified and linear. *We have to put out this fire right now!* For those leaders who feel ill-equipped to handle high-level planning but understand the basics of 'putting out a fire', a crisis offers a reprieve from feelings of inadequacy, and a sense of contribution through simple, honest, hard work. These people may not feel equipped to provide the deeper leadership skills, but if the group can conspire to orchestrate a crisis, they can demonstrate high levels of visible sacrifice as a substitute. The unconscious hope may be that since emotions are high and everyone is watching closely, martyrdom during a crisis will be remembered more vividly by the team and this person's superiors. They may hope to achieve the image of a team member who does what it takes when it really counts.

The Warrior-in-Peacetime archetype fits well in such a climate. Group members who gained accolades and a sense of self-worth on the battlefield may struggle to engage in leadership tasks that are less action-oriented. It is often easier for such individuals to search for another battle, or, failing that, start a fight. This kind of leader may be adept at 'fighting', but unskilled at making meaning of more mundane situations, and thus incapable of crafting and communicating a deeper vision to his/her people that does not involve manufactured drama.

Groups may also leverage crises to salvage member relations, as we discussed previously. Groups tend to band together and set aside intra-group conflict when a salient external threat is presented or engineered. Some part of the group psyche knows this, and may manufacture a crisis as a survival measure when a group's inner relationships are at a breaking point. This can become a habit for the group psyche, and has heavy, obvious drawbacks.

William White (1997) suggests that there is an addictive quality to some organisations' relationship with crisis: 'As with a chemical addiction, there is the phenomenon of building tolerance—it takes crises of greater frequency and magnitude to satiate the need' (p. 60).

As leaders or group facilitators, we would be foolish to take such organisational problems at face value, and focus only on corrective measures for individual components within the system. Until we address the deeper motivations on a systemic level, we will run into entrenched organisational defence mechanisms. Any solution we propose will be thwarted by a psychic workaround.

We can assume that the group unconscious is purposeful and goal-oriented, although it does not share the group's explicitly stated goals.

A group that is subconsciously grateful for crises will fight fiercely to defend the systems that create them.

What is a group caught in crisis compulsion telling us? When we apply our group-as-a-whole understanding, we might guess that these types of groups communicate one or more of the following:

- 'Our leaders feel unclear about how to be effective, so they create situations that are high-urgency and black-and-white'.
- 'We are lacking a compelling vision, so we are struggling to find meaning in the mundane, and a crisis gives us a sense of purpose'.
- 'We have unresolved relational conflict among members that threatens to destroy the group, so we are mobilising an external threat to bring ourselves together'.

It becomes the leader or consultant's job to identify the unspoken narrative that contributes to the crisis compulsion and creatively challenge it. For the first situation above, leadership coaching and expanded training might be prudent. Additionally, it can be helpful to build in a reward structure that recognises desired leadership skills, such as proper planning, delegation, and forward-thinking. For the second situation, upper leadership may need to reconsider the mission statement and how to better connect it to the everyday work of the team. Is it just feel-good fluff, or is it helpful in guiding the everyday experience of organisational members? For the last situation, group mediation, teamwork facilitation, or team restructuring can be starting points.

We can take the above and identify specific risk factors that contribute to organisations falling into crisis compulsion. An organisation prepares the soil for crisis compulsion by hiring or promoting leaders based on narrow skill sets, compliance, agreeableness, and perceived work effort. These may sound reasonable, but consider that a proclivity towards compliance and agreeableness can preclude an individual from exercising discriminatory judgement, a crucial leadership skill. Approval addicts are likely to struggle to make the necessary unpopular decisions. Likewise, the perceived effort put into a job does not necessarily correlate with a job well done. Sometimes, it signals the opposite.

Organisations may be seduced into weighing these qualities favourably in promotional decisions, since they make for a harmonious working environment when the individual is working at a position of lower hierarchical power. The logic is often as simple as, 'This person was great on the assembly line, so they will be great as a shift manager'.

Odysseus, typically lauded for his cleverness and resilience, may actually serve as a paragon of such a leader. He performed well in wartime under King Agamemnon, and was involved with the winning tactic of the Trojan Horse. Yet, his cleverness and boldness did not translate to effective leadership over his men on the journey home. When he was tasked to bring his men safely home, the voyage lasted ten years and all his men perished through the never-ending stream of crises they manifested. Odysseus had a habit of angering the gods and mobilising archetypes to act against his crew. Likewise, many of us may recognise similar tendencies in leaders of today, and perhaps within ourselves as well.

CHAPTER 16

The pain of transformation

The following conversation applies heavily to new leaders, but also has broader implications.

Leadership roles are often sought-after and glorified—or vilified and resented. This polarity implies a strong gravitational force either way, as we discussed in earlier chapters. We think of leadership and power as intertwined. Yet there are ways in which stepping into leadership is heavily disempowering as well.

What is rarely expected by newly appointed leaders is the level of personal alienation, loneliness, and strife with prior peers. Colleagues who served as confidantes can no longer be confided in, as the information a leader attains is often sensitive, and a spotlight on the leadership role means such treatment could be seen as inappropriately preferential. Peers who previously felt at ease sharing in humour and jokes become aware that a new leader's impressions and judgements carry heavier consequences. The equilibrium of the system is disrupted, and the ways that both parties were meeting their relational needs are no longer viable.

The Greek account of Actaeon gives us a feel for the dangers involved with personal transformation in the group context:

Prince Actaeon is out pursuing stag with his hunting party. After a successful morning, he instructs his party to take a break. Actaeon wanders away from the party and finds a cave, where he surprises the goddess Artemis, who is bathing with the aid of her nymphs. They rush to cover her, but it is too late, she has been seen naked by Actaeon. Artemis reaches for her arrows, but they are not at hand, so she splashes water from the bath into Actaeon's eyes, and says 'Now go and tell, if you can, that you have seen Artemis unapparelled'. As he stumbles away, he is transformed into a stag. His hunter's confidence is replaced by fear, yet he cannot help but admire his own new speed.

While he takes stock of his situation, one of his hunting dogs notices him and lets out a cry. The pack pursues him along the familiar course that he has chased many stags in the past, and when they catch him, he is killed by their jaws as his friends cheer them on.

In the story, Actaeon does not see Artemis naked by his own design. He stumbles in by accident. He was quite satisfied in his current station, yet he is unexpectedly filled with the vision of the divine feminine huntress unclothed. There is a transformation that takes place that alters his relation to the natural world—he has become more a part of it. And he has become less a part of his hunting party.

His new appearance makes him a target. His belonging with his peers and dogs is utterly gone through the process of his transformation—they only see him as a trophy to conquer now. He is not one of them anymore. If we return to our Norse creation myth metaphor, Actaeon is moved abruptly to the cold ice of Niflheim in relation to his group. The transformation comes with deeply painful consequences.

Coming from leadership roles in therapeutic organisations, and having witnessed incredible self-transformation on the part of many clients, it is my belief that this story plays out often in this realm. There are reasons why primary mental health treatment centres do not generally recommend that clients return home to the same environment. An oft-cited reason is removing them from the established unhealthy roles and dynamics with friends/family, but another less-recognised reason is held in the Actaeon story: A changed man/woman is apt to be cannibalised or targeted by his prior peers.

There is a documentary titled *The Work* (2017) in which a men's-work-focused organisation enters Folsom Prison to do therapeutic-style processes with a subpopulation of the inmates. I was told by an administrator for the Mankind Project that the men who participate in this practice have to be permanently separated from the general population prisoners after participating, because they are targeted by the other inmates if they return. Personal transformation—an experience of Artemis—is both deeply valuable, and also leaves one extremely vulnerable to the malice of one's past peers. That experience of divine feminine may mark these men to be hunted.

Likewise, when I have coached newly promoted leaders, a common theme is loneliness and alienation. Where there was previously community, trust, and respect, old colleagues now hold a distance. Suspicion, distrust, and any other projections that are held in the system towards those in power are likely to surface. These new leaders are often times and without warning stripped of their support network. It is not uncommon for new leaders to fantasise about a return to less responsibility, as discussed previously in the leadership chapter.

Interestingly, in the spring of 2023, the US Surgeon General claimed that loneliness causes health detriment equal to smoking fifteen cigarettes per day (Seltz, 2023). In my experience, it is rare that higher-up leaders grasp this and offer extra support to newly promoted managers, even though many upper-level leaders have experienced something similar.

CHAPTER 17

Collision of paradigms: Isomorphism vs projection

When we speak about projection at a group level, we understand that an individual or subgroup is made to hold psychic archetypal energy that belongs to the whole group. This frees up others from having to act out this energy.

Yet the exact opposite idea is also embraced by intelligent thinkers as well, such as the family clinician Dr Tony Issenmann. *Isomorphism* refers to a system replicating patterns across different levels of its hierarchy. As above, so below. This concept predicts that interrelational conflicts among company owners, for example, would find a way to play out similarly at lower management levels. We see this in the Arthurian Fisher King myth after the king endures a thigh wound. While the king is wounded, the whole kingdom languishes. Similarly, when Set steals the Egyptian throne from Osiris, the land and people suffer. And when the Shinto sun goddess Amaterasu is forced into the cave, her realm is left in chaos.

So which is it? Do groups project archetypal energy onto individuals and subgroups, or are the same patterns played out over different levels?

It is possible that there is room for both phenomena. Each might occur at different times and under different conditions.

113

Sometimes groups may delegate psychic shadow material as projections, and sometimes groups may act out such material across different levels. I can think of examples of both from my own experience within wilderness therapy organisations, and even both phenomena within the same organisation simultaneously.

I recall an anxious director who seemed driven by a fear of failure. The narrative that they shared about the company's history revolved around certain old partners-turned-villains, who were waiting in the wing with sharpened knives for the company to falter. Their particular flavour of anxiety seemed to permeate to the therapist team, who became preoccupied with pleasing outside business referral sources at the expense of work quality. Of course, a strong sense of customer service is important in a healthy business, but when anxiety reshapes value priority, there is a damaging pattern present. In this case, it appeared that the anxiety at one level (the director) had bled into another level (the clinical team), and then from there to management, etc.

Yet at the same time, in the same organisation, there was a strong tendency to scapegoat. Private conversations with the executive often involved open blaming of certain therapists or managers, with the subject of such vitriol changing on a weekly basis. There seemed to be a perpetual search for the problem within the organisation. It felt like a game of hot-potato or musical chairs at times.

Behind closed doors, middle managers reported feelings of relief when the weekly blame was assigned to someone else. Middle managers openly talked among themselves about their strategy for moving out of the blame spotlight. Using our group-as-a-whole lens, it appeared that the organisation hoped to place its incompetence into one vessel, as we discussed in the scapegoating chapter. Thus, it seems possible for groups to display isomorphism, projective identification, both, or neither, depending on the context.

Isomorphism seems less likely to occur when a leader is holding a strong archetypal role in the system. In cults such as the Osho's, for example, when a guru sits at the top of the hierarchy, it seems less likely that other members will be celebrated for their own wisdom. Osho's second-in-command held something different for the system, as she was organised, strategic, and brutal.

It is as though sometimes we ask our leaders to hold an archetype for us that we do not feel comfortable embodying, and at other times we ask them to model an archetype with which we wish to establish more contact. In systems embodying the latter, we can imagine a child looking up to the parents, and imitating the behaviour they see, even when it is unhealthy or abusive.

Another idea is that within different subgroups in an organisation, each archetype must find a home, and since there exists a model for archetypal expression at one level, this becomes the default expression in subgroups. This might help us answer the question, 'How does isomorphism serve the group?' In this case, perhaps it is by providing a template for archetypal expression.

A third idea is that the piece being enacted at different levels is especially important, and the group is acting out this material isomorphically in an attempt to resolve or integrate it. The unconscious is a powerful force, and in such a case would recruit all levels of an organisation in an attempt to either integrate repressed material or otherwise meet its desires by playing out a dynamic.

CHAPTER 18

Grief and adjourning

We opened the book with a myth for the forming stage of groups, and it is appropriate that we close with a myth for adjourning. An implication of Tuckman's model is that groups have a life cycle, and any life cycle must include death. In my experience, the group psyche tends to place a high emphasis on group survival and be strangely resilient to threats of group dissolution, much like a living organism. Yet, like living organisms, resilience for groups has limits. Adjourning is the final of Tuckman's stages of group development, and like death, typically evokes feelings of grief.

Groups can adjourn in a graceful manner after a desired goal is accomplished, or the process can be premature and messy. For the latter, there can be many factors leading to an unsatisfying group death: internal dynamics, external forces, leadership failures, etc. William White (1997) attributes organisational existential crises or 'breakups' to impermeable boundaries that develop, and the unsustainable pressures on members that result.

Grieving is a process we associate with loss, and the adjourning of a group always involves a loss. Adjourning typically refers to the whole group disbanding, but we might also consider that any change to group membership, whether losing or gaining, represents the death of the group as it was, and that any such change is likely to induce the grieving process to some extent.

The extent of melancholy that invades groups upon the loss of a member can be surprising. This holds true even when the departed member was toxic. Groups sometimes viciously scapegoat a member, only to refer to them fondly once they are absent. Remaining group members might tell grandiose, exaggerated stories of the departed member's deeds and relationships. A fondness that was not present before may arise. Therefore, wise leaders should never expect gratitude for actively eliminating a toxic member. Many managers likely learn this the hard way when they make firing decisions to benefit their team.

We can look to the evolutionary significance of group death as a partial explainer. Historically, there was safety in groups, in an otherwise hostile world. This added safety often existed even if some of the members were relatively undesirable as teammates. Group members who otherwise felt solid in their group identity can at some level become troubled when confronted with the mutability and impermanence of their group.

The affection that groups find for ex-members also breathes life into the idea that each member holds something of the group's psyche, and that something of an identity crisis occurs when a member leaves. As we have discussed, the departure of a member who held negative projections necessitates either a new vehicle for these projections, or a reintegration of the shadow material that this person held.

A member's departure is a crucial moment, as discussed in the scapegoating section, since it forces this choice to the group. The group psyche needs to have a home for all parts of itself, or no equilibrium can be had. The group will feel a shared sense of anxiety if it is unable to find a suitable container for a projection and is resistant to integrating the material. This is the dilemma that faces a group with changing membership, a modified adjourning phase.

In general, the adjourning stage can pair with myths about end times.

In the Norse pantheon, the gods are aware of their future annihilation, an apocalyptic event known as Ragnarök. Odin is building up his cache of brave warriors in Asgard throughout his reign in preparation. It is prophesied that the gods will perish when the giants and demons rise up against them, in a great battle that will result in the stars and sky collapsing, and the earth sinking into the sea. Afterwards, a being known as the Nameless One will give birth to the world anew.

In Norse mythology, it is said that the last fight will take place on a vast battlefield called Vigrid. A theme within this future battle is mutual destruction. Thor and the Midgard Serpent will kill each other, as will Loki and Heimdall. The god Tyr will slay Garm, the dog of Niflheim, but be clawed to death in return.

Mutual destruction, which hints at both murder and pairing, might be a special case. It suggests an interconnectedness of certain energies, where the existence or loss of one is tied to the other.

For example, the Norse god Tyr presides over legal matters, and we could associate him with boundaries. Garm, on the other hand, is the wild avatar of the icy north. We recall that the frozen north can represent total individuality, a complete rejection of the joining process (whereas the fiery south represents the complete absorption of identity by the group).

Of course, group boundaries have a strong and potentially contentious relationship with individuality. To accept group norms is to lose some freedom as an individual. The boundaries of Tyr maintain the group's integrity, at the expense of Garm's individuality. So we should not be surprised that Tyr and Garm are at odds in the myth. The prophecy of Ragnarök suggests that the conflict between the two is an ongoing existential threat to groups, such that when balance is not found, it may lead to end times for the group. Group boundaries must be shaped to allow for some preservation of individuality, if a group is to survive.

It is not uncommon that groups entering the adjourning phase will manufacture conflict. Conflict can be a welcome distraction from feelings of grief, and may even allow for the group psyche to devalue the group, thus minimising the impact of the loss. This is similar to what we might see from a child moving away from a close friend, who starts a fight in order to avoid a painful goodbye. Skilled group facilitators might choose to name this aloud to a group, which can help preserve member relationships and encourage processing of the feelings in the room.

As for grieving, King Priam of Troy gives us something of a template:

> Towards the end of the Trojan War, Achilles kills Hector in a duel outside the city gates. Achilles ties the corpse behind his chariot and trails it back to his camp, where it is disrespected and dragged about for eleven days. Yet Hector's body does not decay, because it is protected by Apollo.
>
> King Priam, in pain over his son Hector's death, sneaks behind Greek lines with the help of Hermes to ransom the body. Priam reaches Achilles, who treats him with courtesy, as Achilles is reminded of his own father. Achilles accepts the ransom, and Priam is able to take Hector's body back to Troy for a cremation.

In a society devoted to perpetuating comfort, grieving can be an intimidating and alien proposition. It is seductive to sink into distractions, and groups will often do just that in order to avoid the hard feelings that come with contemplating adjourning.

When we avoid mourning, we push Hector's body away to be held by the Greeks. Groups that do this prolong their agony, staying stuck in the part of our story where Hector's preserved body is dragged along by Achilles. This is a kind of limbo, or purgatory. That which is not mourned lingers and haunts. Some groups (and cultures) spend years here, or never leave. Wounds cannot heal, nor can the body decompose fully. It is stuck in-between.

It takes courage to face grief. Proper grieving requires stepping into the darkness and crossing a threshold, as Priam does. We do not move into true grieving if we stay within the city gates. We must retrieve Hector, be close to the body, and honour him. Hector's body is not recovered through inaction. Especially in a culture with so many distractions, Hector does not come to us, we move to him.

As a coach, therapist, or group facilitator, often this means observing the experienced loss, and inviting conversation about it—an act which will often elicit group defence mechanisms. There is no simple hack for holding the grief space for a group, but a tender and empathetic touch is helpful. It is a time to set down Hercules and invite Persephone energy.

Lastly, we know from experience that not all group adjournings are equal. A happy departure after a successful project completion is much preferred to unceremonious disbanding after some sort of failure. Sometimes external factors create conditions for group failure, but often, and even in the presence of favourable outside conditions, internal group dynamics play a large role in manifesting failure.

We have touched on many ways that groups may sabotage themselves or recruit toxic dynamics to serve an unconscious agenda. When such forces run rampant, there can be a real threat to the group's survival, even though we assume that the unconscious always intends for group survival.

These groups devour themselves, much like the snake manifestation of Crom Cruach in Moore and Twomey's film *The Secret of Kells* (2009) (Crom Cruach was a pagan god whose name translates to 'crooked and bloody'). We are reminded of the Ouroboros snake from Egyptian myth that eats its own tail. The Ouroboros is often thought to symbolise rebirth, yet serpentine also can mean 'sly and tempting', which speaks to the seductive quality of undermining, unconscious forces in groups. In Norse mythology, the Midgard Serpent circles the Earth and holds its tail in its mouth. It is said that when it releases it, this will trigger Ragnarök. Also in Norse mythology is Níðhöggr, a serpent who gnaws at the roots of the World Tree, so there is a sense that the serpent is an eroding force.

For a real-life example of 'the snake eating itself', we might consider Solzhenitsyn's *Gulag Archipelago*. Individuals and groups who helped the communist regime rise to power are eventually also arrested for imagined offences. No one is safe. The snake destructively eats itself.

CHAPTER 19

Here-and-now work for us as a culture

There is much more to discuss regarding the intersection of mythology and group dynamics. Yet our ambition with this work is to open a door, not explore the full territory. To this end, we hope to provide closure to the book by interpreting some of our societal patterns, and to offer a different orientation.

In some versions of Greek myth, Nemesis is the one to lure Narcissus to his reflection in the pool, and ultimately his death, as he becomes transfixed by his own imagined beauty and dies staring at his own reflection. Our culture is mobilising Nemesis against the narcissistic elements within our own culture. The narcissistic elements hold no consideration for the other and elevate themselves inappropriately. We see a dark narcissism present in stories such as Harvey Weinstein's and Bill Cosby's. It is right that these energies be confronted. And yet there is a productive path forward, and also many ways we might become lost in the woods.

As individuals, we can say that each of us is a microcosm of society as a whole. We all contain within our psyches a Nemesis, a Narcissus, a Tyrant, a Warrior, a Lover, a Criminal, a Victim, an Innocent Child, a Bully, a Mentor, and so forth. All elements of society are mirrored within each of our psyches. Kahlil Gibran said, 'In one drop of water are found all the secrets of all the oceans; in one aspect of You are found all the aspects of existence'. A good therapist moves a client towards the integration of these inner personalities, such that the person moves towards wholeness. That is to say, the healthiest among us are no longer repressing as many parts of ourselves. Fewer rooms of our own inner houses remain off-limits when this work has been done. Our psyches become explored territory, to an ever-increasing extent.

Competent therapists know that this process requires moving away from the shaming response, and granting some intentional amnesty to the scary parts of ourselves. We can't integrate shadow material that we are unwilling to first accept. This process shouldn't happen willy-nilly, but rather at an appropriate pace in which our consciousness can metabolise what we find in a manner that preserves our grounded sense of self. This is not to say we teach ourselves to condone the harmful parts of ourselves. As Nathaniel Branden writes, we can accept something about ourselves to be true without endorsing it. Acknowledgement is a crucial first step towards personal evolution.

As a group system, society may do well to mirror this process. As mentioned previously, when Nelson Mandela took over in South Africa, he granted some amnesty to individuals who testified to crimes and atrocities that had occurred during Apartheid. He saw it as important to know the extent of the systemic awfulness. Moving forward, this was more important than exacting retribution and enforcing punishments.

In essence, he took away the shaming and individual blame, and took a systems approach. He wanted to bring the crimes out into the open, out of the subconscious of the group, and shine a light on them. This is required for integration. This does mean that some individuals *get away with it* to some extent, as measured by our normal fantasies for punitive justice—and this is understandably hard to swallow. We may have to choose: Do we want revenge, or do we want to build a healthier system for the future? Investing in the future may require that we prioritise integration of our group psyche rather than engage in the satisfaction of retribution. This is not the same as turning a blind eye to the corruption of those who were involved; it is closer to the opposite. We need to find a way to take a full look.

As well-intentioned and important as newer movements such as 'Time's Up' and 'Defund the Police' are, we might also ask ourselves if the methods employed bring more to light or push more into the psychic underworld. It is clear that toxic elements infect the power structure and there is a need for change. History has also shown that crucifixion is typically ineffective for producing positive, lasting social change in the direction intended by the crucifiers.

In short, shadow-shaming, or 'callout culture', is ineffective for instilling real healthy change in groups. This has proven true when working with therapeutic populations in organisations, and it is true in a more universal way. Accepting shadow material is necessary for integration.

This is different than affirming toxic behaviour or being passively permissive towards bad actors. We can and should see the darkness for what it is. It is our cultural fetish for heavy-handed shaming that we could do without. Psychological theory and group relations work inform us that shaming and aggressive counter-persecution merely displace and perpetuate suffering in the system.

The group-as-a-whole work leads us to the conclusion that bottling up the bad within certain individuals and slicing them away does not work to improve the group situation in the long run. As our colleague Jason Clemares says, 'The bad just won't go away'. It is in us somewhere, and moving forward as a culture is more about bringing it up into the light and integrating those expressions of ourselves rather than shoving them away into the darkness. In *The Gulag Archipelago*, Aleksandr Solzhenitsyn (2007) writes,

> If only it were all so simple! If only there were evil people some-where insidiously committing evil deeds, and it was necessary only to separate them from the rest of us and destroy them. But the line dividing good and evil cuts through the heart of every human being. (p. 168)

Such a shift is not a full solution, merely an appropriate starting point for a healing process. We can also apply the here-and-now group per-spective to the increasing polarisation of global politics. What is it doing for the group-as-a-whole to enact such a division? According to some accounts of the Trojan War, Zeus planned to use the conflict as a way of eradicating mankind. Perhaps there is a Zeus energy within us that longs for destruction. It would certainly fit into the theme of shame.

Nathaniel Branden (1995) writes that when we carry deep shame or regret, self-punishment and self-sabotage become tools we use to set the scale right. It will feel unbearable for someone carrying deep shame to experience great success—they do not believe they are worthy, and will find a way to sabotage it. Part of this has to do with control, perhaps, since this person believes that failure is what is deserved, so it will come eventually, and it is better to descend on one's own terms. Basically, we find nuanced ways to reproduce our internal story about ourselves on the external stage.

We can guess that an identical phenomenon might occur in groups. It is not difficult to pinpoint sources of shame for our culture: In the West, we can point to the awful treatment of indigenous communities, the history of slavery, and current environmental destruction. Of course there is a deep shame that comes with this for the group psyche. We carry this somewhere, whether we attempt to externalise the blame or not.

Robert Bly (1990) writes about *katabasis* in *Iron John*, the psychological descent into suffering that is often a precursor for growth. It certainly feels that the Western culture in a stage of descent in many ways. Divorce rates are high, depression is rampant, addiction is entrenched, racial tensions have re-emerged, and environmental damage is profound. Apocalyptic themes are commonplace in our cinema, reflecting the fantasies and fears that preoccupy our group consciousness.

In the early 2020s, it feels as if the themes highlighted in this text are especially significant on a cultural level. There are signs of groupthink, a fight reaction on a societal level, metaphorical and literal murder. Riots and bold accusations between different sects threaten to widen the relational gap between those with different ideologies. Each side has its heroes and gods.

Within each of the political parties, certain projections seem to be especially tempting. If the left can hold our weakness and naïveté, those of us on the right can live out our fantasy of being strong, capable, and independent. If the right can hold our rigidity and inner tyrant, then we on the left can live our liberal fantasy of being enlightened, serene, and nurturing. In both camps, there is a sense of something being pushed away. We recall our earlier discussion on Hercules and Persephone.

In both of the above examples, we attempt to flee via transcendence, as Icarus does in myth. In the story, Icarus and his father make wings from wax and feathers to escape their imprisonment in an island tower, absconding through the air. During the escape, an ecstatic Icarus flies too high, not heeding his father's warnings, and the sun melts the wax in his wings, sending him down into the ocean to die. The thinking is this: If we can just gain enough virtue, perhaps we can rise above into enlightenment and avoid the dirty mundane parts of ourselves. Bly (1990) discusses this on an individual level in adolescent boys, but we see it in other groups as well, prevalent in today's social media sphere. Bly calls this expression of the archetype the *flying boy*.

As in the myth, flight away from something often sends us right back to it. Had Icarus stayed closer to the oceanic waters instead of forcing himself far away into perilous heights, he might have maintained his flight. Again, water in myth is thought to represent the unconscious, so it is fitting that Icarus' attempts to distance himself from the ocean brought him back to it in dramatic fashion. When we try to escape from the murky depths of ourselves, they rush back at us with sometimes lethal force.

This myth is alive in those who disown their own inner racist while loudly denouncing the slightest offences by others. They may voraciously proclaim themselves allies of the cause. Rarely is there a sense of real ownership for the biases they themselves carry. The myth tells us that by flying too far from the dark, frothy water, we will likely end up drowning in it. Diving into the darkness is messy work, but necessary for real integration of the fractured collective self. Dr Simon Western urges us to 'stick with the trouble', and it is our hope that the use of mythic metaphor represents another tool for change agents who wish to do so.

References

Bates, D., Ogilvie, M., & Pole, E. (2016). Occupy: In theory and practice. *Critical Discourse Studies, 13*(3): 341–355.

Bennis, W. G. (1976). *Unconscious Conspiracy: Why Leaders Can't Lead.* New York: AMACOM.

Bierlein, J. F. (1995). *Parallel Myths.* New York: Ballantine.

Bion, W. R. (1959). *Experiences in Groups, and Other Papers.* London: Tavistock.

Bly, R. (1986). *A Little Book on the Human Shadow.* Memphis: Raccoon Books, Inc. [HarperOne, 1988]

Bly, R. (1990). *Iron John: A Book About Men.* Boston, MA: Addison-Wesley [Rider, 2001]

Bly, R. (1997). *The Sibling Society: An Impassioned Call for the Rediscovery of Adulthood.* Boston, MA: Addison-Wesley.

Branden, N. (1995). *Six Pillars of Self-Esteem: The Definitive Work on Self-Esteem by the Leading Pioneer in the Field.* New York: Bantam.

Britannica (2024, March 7). Isis. Retrieved from https://www.britannica.com/topic/Isis-Egyptian-goddess

Bulfinch, T. (2004). *Bulfinch's Mythology.* New York: Modern Library.

Campbell, J. (1949). *The Hero with a Thousand Faces.* New York: Pantheon. [New World Library, 2012]

Cayley, D. (2019). *The Ideas of René Girard: An Anthropology of Religion and Violence*. Independently published.

Crimi, S. (2021). From pharmakon to pharmakós: Inverted scapegoating during the 'Covid pandemic'. *Hermes Runs the Game: Myth, Sacrifice and Initiation*. Retrieved from https://www.academia.edu/51372759/From_Pharmakon_to_Pharmak%C3%B3s_Inverted_Scapegoating_During_the_covid_pandemic_

De Mello, A., & Stroud, J. F. (1990). *Awareness: A Conversation with the Masters*. London: Image. [Image, 1992]

De Waal, F. (2005). *Our Inner Ape*. New York: Riverhead Books.

Edinger, E. F. (1994). *The Eternal Drama: The Inner Meaning of Greek Mythology*. Boston, MA: Shambhala. [Shambhala, 2013]

Ferry, D. (1993). *Gilgamesh: A New Rendering in English Verse*. New York: Farrar, Straus & Giroux.

Frazer, J. G. (1922). *The Golden Bough: A Study in Magic and Religion*. London: Palgrave Macmillan. [Macmillan, 1990]

Freud, S. (1921b). *Group Psychology and the Analysis of the Ego*. S. E., 18: 67–134. London: Hogarth.

Gabriel, Y., & Hampton, M. (1999). *Organizations in Depth: The Psychoanalysis of Organizations*. London: SAGE.

Janis, I. L. (1997). Groupthink. *Psychology Today*, November 1971. Available at: https://www.psychologytoday.com/intl/basics/groupthink

Jung, C. G. (1969). *Collected Works of C.G. Jung, Volume 9 (Part 2): Aion: Researches into the Phenomenology of the Self*. New York: Princeton University Press.

Jung, C. G. (1971). *Collected Works of C.G. Jung, Volume 6: Psychological Types*. New York: Princeton University Press.

Jung, C. G. (1991). *The Archetypes and the Collective Unconscious* (2nd edn). London: Routledge.

Karpman, S. B. (1968). Fairy tales and script drama analysis. *Transactional Analysis Bulletin, 7*(26): 39–43.

Klein, M. (1946). Notes on some schizoid mechanisms. *The Journal of Psychotherapy Practice and Research, 5*(2): 160–179.

Lacan, J. (2016). *The Sinthome: The Seminar of Jacques Lacan, Book XXIII*. Cambridge: Polity Press.

Lencioni, P. (2002). *The Five Dysfunctions of a Team: A Leadership Fable* (20th anniversary edn). San Francisco, CA: Jossey-Bass.

The Lumineers (2012). Stubborn love (song). In: *The Lumineers*. Dualtone Records.

Moore, R., & Gillette, D. (1992). *King Warrior Magician Lover: Rediscovering the Archetypes of the Mature Masculine* (new edn). San Francisco, CA: Bravo.

Moxnes, P. (1999). Deep roles: Twelve primordial roles of mind and organization. *Human Relations*, *52*(11): 1427–1444. https://doi.org/10.1177/001872679905201104

Obholzer, A., & Roberts, V. Z. (Eds.) (2019). *The Unconscious at Work: A Tavistock Approach to Making Sense of Organizational Life*. Abingdon: Routledge.

Peterson, J. (Host). (2014, 29 March). 2014 Personality Lecture 20: Conscientiousness (Biology & Traits) [Video lecture]. In: *Personality and its Transformations* (Lecture Series). Jordan B. Peterson (YouTube Channel).

Plotkin, B., & Berry, T. (2003). *Soulcraft: Crossing into the Mysteries of Nature and Psyche*. Novato, CA: New World Library.

Schwartz, H. S. (1997). Psychodynamics of political correctness. *The Journal of Applied Behavioral Science*, *33*(2): 132–148. https://doi.org/10.1177/0021886397332003

The Secret of Kells (2009). Directed by Tomm Moore & Nora Twomey. Les Armateurs, Vivi Film, Cartoon Saloon.

Seltz, A. (2023, May 2). Loneliness poses risks as deadly as smoking: Surgeon General. *AP News*. https://apnews.com/article/surgeon-general-loneliness-334450f7bb5a77e88d8085b178340e19 (last accessed 22 June 2023).

Solzhenitsyn, A. I. (2007). *The Gulag Archipelago, 1918–1956: Volume 1: An Experiment in Literary Investigation*. New York: Harper Perennial.

Stahl, G. K., Maznevski, M. L., Voigt, A., & Jonsen, K. (2010). Unraveling the effects of cultural diversity in teams: A meta-analysis of research on multicultural work groups. *Journal of International Business Studies*, *41*(4): 690–709. https://doi.org/10.1057/jibs.2009.85

Stokoe, P. (2021). Application of psychoanalytic concepts. In: M. Sher & D. Lawlor (Ed.), *An Introduction to Systems Psychodynamics* (pp. 80–93). Abingdon, Oxon: Routledge, 2022.

Storr, W. (2019). *The Science of Storytelling: Why Stories Make Us Human and How To Tell Them Better*. Glasgow: William Collins.

Tuckman, B. W. (1965). Developmental sequence in small groups. *Psychological Bulletin*, *63*(6): 384–399. https://doi.org/10.1037/h0022100

Vaughan, D. (2016). *The Challenger Launch Decision: Risky Technology, Culture, and Deviance at NASA, Enlarged Edition*. Chicago, IL: University of Chicago Press.

Vazard, J. (2022). Feeling the unknown: Emotions of uncertainty and their valence. *Erkenntnis*. https://doi.org/10.1007/s10670-022-00583-1

Western, S. (2017). Where's Daddy? Integrating the paternal and maternal stance to deliver non-authoritarian leadership for the network society. *Organisational and Social Dynamics, 17*(2): 198–221.

Westervelt, W. D. (1910). *Legends of Maui: A Demi God of Polynesia and of His Mother Hina*. Honolulu, HI: The Hawaiian Gazette.

White, W. L. (1997). *The Incestuous Workplace: Stress and Distress in the Organizational Family*. Minneapolis, MN: Hazelden.

Woodman, M. (1998). *Sitting by the Well: Bringing the Feminine to Consciousness Through Language, Dreams, and Metaphor*. Boulder, CO: Sounds True.

The Work (2017). Directed by Jairus McLeary & Gethin Aldous. Blanket Fort Media.

Index